Effects of Substance Abuse Treatment on AIDS Risk Behaviors

Effects of Substance Abuse Treatment on AIDS Risk Behaviors has been co-published simultaneously as *Journal of Addictive Diseases*, Volume 17, Number 4 1998.

The *Journal of Addictive Diseases* Monographic "Separates"
(formerly *Advances in Alcohol & Substance Abuse* series)*

Below is a list of "separates," which in serials librarianship means a special issue simultaneously
   published as a special journal issue or double-issue and as a "separate" hardbound monograph. (This
   is a format which we also call a "Docuserial.")

"Separates" are published because specialized libraries or professionals may wish to purchase a
   specific thematic issue by itself in a format which can be separately cataloged and shelved, as
   opposed to purchasing the journal on an on-going basis. Faculty members may also more easily
   consider a "separate" for classroom adoption.

"Separates" are carefully classified separately with the major book jobbers so that the journal tie-in
   can be noted on new book order slips to avoid duplicate purchasing.

You may wish to visit the Haworth's website at . . .

http://www.haworthpressinc.com

. . . to search our online catalog for complete tables of contents of these separates and related
publications.

You may also call 1-800-HAWORTH (outside US/Canada: 607-722-5857), or Fax 1-800–895-0582
(outside US/Canada: 607-771-0012), or e-mail at:

getinfo@haworthpressinc.com

Smoking and Illicit Drug Use, edited by Mark S. Gold, MD (JAD 17(1), 1998.
Available now.) *"Based on an understanding of the brain biology of reward,
Gold and his colleagues provide policymakers, clinicians, and the public with
the best-ever look at the reason why 90% of the nation's more than 60 million
cigarette smokers want to quit but have trouble achieving that life-saving
goal." (Robert L. DuPont, MD, President, Institute for Behavior and Health,
and Professor of Psychiatry, Georgetown University School of Medicine,
Rockville, MD) Focuses on the addictive properties of the numerous
constituents of tobacco smoke and nicotine dependency*

***The Integration of Pharmacological and Nonpharmacological Treatments in
Drug/Alcohol Addictions***, edited by Norman S. Miller, MD, and Barry
Stimmel, MD (JAD 16(4), 1997.) *Summarizes and provides the groundwork for
future considerations in developing and integrating medications with the
standard of care for addictions treatment.*

Intensive Outpatient Treatment for the Addictions, edited by Edward Gottheil,
MD, PhD (JAD 16(2), 1997.) *"An invaluable source of up-to-date information
on important issues relating to IOP, including the active ingredients of
successful IOP, the effectiveness of IOP, causes of early dropout, and the
impact of psychiatric status and motivation for change on outcomes for
patients." (Stephen Magura, PhD, Director, Institute for Treatment Research,
National Development & Research institutes, Inc., New York)*

The Neurobiology of Cocaine Addiction: From Bench to Bedside, edited by
Herman Joseph, PhD, and Barry Stimmel, MD (JAD 15(4), 1997.) *"Provides*

an excellent overview of advances in the treatment of cocaine addiction." (The Annals of Pharmacotherapy)

The Effectiveness of Social Interventions for Homeless Substance Abusers, edited by Gerald J. Stahler, PhD, and Barry Stimmel, MD (JAD 14(4), 1996.) *"Any policymaker or administrator seeking to have a positive impact on the complex problems of this population would be well-advised to thoroughly digest the contents of this volume." (Journal of Behavioral Health Services & Research (formerly the Journal of Mental Health Administration))*

Experimental Therapeutics in Addiction Medicine, edited by Stephen Magura, PhD, and Andrew Rosenblum, PhD (JAD 13(3/4), 1995.) *"Recommended for any clinician involved in caring for patients with substance abuse problems and for those interested in furthering research in this discipline." (The Annals of Pharmacotherapy)*

Comorbidity of Addictive and Psychiatric Disorders, edited by Norman S. Miller, MD (JAD 12(3), 1993.) *"A wealth of factual information . . . IT SHOULD BE INCLUDED IN THE LIBRARY OF EVERY PSYCHIATRIC HOSPITAL BECAUSE IT IS AN EXCELLENT REFERENCE BOOK." (Israel Journal of Psychiatry)*

Cocaine: Physiological and Physiopathological Effects, edited by Alfonso Paredes, MD, and David A. Gorlick, MD, PhD (JAD 11(4), 1993.) *"The broad range of psychiatric and medical consequences of the epidemic of cocaine use described in this volume should jolt everyone toward increasing strategies to educate, motivate, and stimulate health practitioners at all levels." (Perspectives on Addictions Nursing)*

What Works in Drug Abuse Epidemiology, edited by Blanche Frank, PhD, and Ronald Simeone, PhD (JAD 11(1), 1992. Softcover available November 1995.) *"An excellent reference text not only for researchers and scholars, but also for administrators, policymakers, law enforcements agents, and health educators who value the importance of research in decisionmaking at both the micro and macro levels of the ever-growing substance abuse speciality." (International Journal of Epidemiology)*

Cocaine, AIDS, and Intravenous Drug Use, edited by Samuel R. Friedman, PhD, and Douglas S. Lipton, PhD (JAD 10(4), 1991.) *"EXAMINES WHAT HAS BEEN SUCCESSFUL IN TREATMENT AND PREVENTION and raises issues to promote greater research in the fields for improved treatment and prevention of drug abuse and HIV-infection." (Sci-Tech Book News)*

Addiction Potential of Abused Drugs and Drug Classes, edited by Carlton K. Erikson, PhD, Martin A. Javors, PhD, and William W. Morgan, PhD (AASA 9(1/2) 1990.) *"A GOOD REFERENCE BOOK FOR ANYONE WHO WORKS IN THE DRUG ABUSE FIELD, particularly those who have responsibilities in the area of community education." (Journal of Psychoactive Drugs)*

Alcohol Research from Bench to Bedside, edited by Enoch Gordis, MD, Boris Tabakoff, PhD, and Markku Linnoila, MD, PhD (AASA 7(3/4), 1989.) *Scientists* *and clinicians examine the exciting endeavors in science that have produced medical knowledge applicable to a wide spectrum of treatment and prevention efforts.*

AIDS and Substance Abuse, edited by Larry Siegel, MD (AASA 7(2), 1988.) *"Contributes in a worthwhile fashion to a number of debates." (British Journal of Addiction)*

Pharmacological Issues in Alcohol and Substance Abuse, edited by Barry Stimmel, MD (AASA 7(1), 1988.) *"GOOD REFERENCE BOOK FOR THE KNOWLEDGE OF THE PHARMACOLOGY OF CERTAIN DRUGS USED IN TREATING CHEMICALLY DEPENDENT CASES." (Anthony B. Radcliffe, MD, Physician in Charge, Chemical Recovery Program, Kaiser, Pontana, California)*

Children of Alcoholics, edited by Margaret Bean-Bayog, MD, and Barry Stimmel, MD (AASA 6(4), 1988.) *"This comprehensive volume EXAMINES SIGNIFICANT RESEARCH AND CLINICAL DEVELOPMENT IN THIS AREA." (T.H.E. Journal)*

Cocaine: Pharmacology, Addiction, and Therapy, edited by Mark S. Gold, MD, Marc Galanter, MD, and Barry Stimmel, MD (AASA 6(2), 1987.) *"DIAGNOSIS AND TREATMENT METHODS ARE ALSO EXPLORED IN THIS HIGHLY USEFUL AND INFORMATIVE BOOK." (Journal of the American Association of Psychiatric Administrators)*

Alcohol and Substance Abuse in Women and Children, edited by Barry Stimmel, MD (AASA 5(3), 1986.) *Here is a timely volume that examines the problems of substance abuse in women and children, with a particular emphasis on the role played by the family in the development and perpetuation of the problem.*

Controversies in Alcoholism and Substance Abuse, edited by Barry Stimmel, MD (AASA 5(1/2), 1986.) *"Thorough, well-informed, and up-to-date." (The British Journal of Psychiatry)*

Alcohol and Substance Abuse in Adolescence, edited by Judith S. Brook, EdD, Dan Lettieri, PhD, David W. Brook, MD, and Barry Stimmel, MD (AASA 4(3/4), 1985.) *"Contains considerable information that would be USEFUL TO MENTAL HEALTH CLINICIANS AND PRIMARY CARE PHYSICIANS WHO DEAL EXTENSIVELY WITH ADOLESCENTS." (The New England Journal of Medicine)*

Alcohol and Drug Abuse in the Affluent, edited by Barry Stimmel, MD (AASA 4(2), 1984.) *"A valuable contribution to drug abuse literature presenting data on a hitherto under-researched population of drug users." (British Journal of Addiction)*

Cultural and Sociological Aspects of Alcoholism and Substance Abuse, edited by Barry Stimmel, MD (AASA 4(1), 1984.) *Experts explore the relationship of* *such factors as ethnicity, family, religion, and gender to chemical abuse and address important implications for treatment.*

Dual Addiction: Pharmacological Issues in the Treatment of Concomitant Alcoholism and Drug Abuse, edited by Mary Jeanne Kreek, MD, and Barry Stimmel, MD (AASA 3(4), 1984.) *"Provides a good overview of dual addiction." (Contemporary Psychology)*

Conceptual Issues in Alcoholism and Substance Abuse, edited by Joyce H. Lowinson, MD, and Barry Stimmel, MD (AASA 3(3), 1984.) *This timely volume emphasizes the relevance of current, basic research to the clinical management of the substance abuser.*

The Addictive Behaviors, edited by Howard Shaffer, PhD, and Barry Stimmel, MD (AASA 3(1/2), 1984.) *"Remarkable . . . is the book's capacity to illustrate social myths and models, to challenge them, and to direct substance abuse professionals in their clinical and research inquiries." (Journal of Psychoactive Drugs)*

Psychosocial Constructs of Alcoholism and Substance Abuse, edited by Barry Stimmel, MD (AASA 2(4), 1983.) *"An excellent vehicle for orienting interested readers toward critical reference materials and important psychosocial issues." (Bulletin of the Society of Psychologists in Addictive Behaviors)*

Federal Priorities in Funding Alcohol and Drug Abuse Programs, edited by Barry Stimmel, MD (AASA 2(3), 1983.) *Reveals and evaluates current federal funding for chemical abuse treatment problems.*

Current Controversies in Alcoholism, edited by Barry Stimmel, MD (AASA 2(2), 1983.) *"Articles vary from reports of sophisticated research to essays backed by thorough literature reviews." (Choice)*

Evaluation of Drug Treatment Programs, edited by Barry Stimmel, MD (AASA 2(1), 1983.) *"Provides the reader with a unique perspective on the effectiveness of drug treatment programs." (American Journal of Pharmaceutical Education)*

Behavioral and Biochemical Issues in Substance Abuse, edited by Frank R. George, PhD, and Doris Clouet, PhD (AASA 10(1/2), 1991.) *"AN EXCELLENT OVERVIEW OF THE POWER OF GENETIC EXPERIMENTAL DESIGNS, the results that can be generated as well as the cautions that must be observed in this approach." (Contemporary Psychology)*

Effects of Maternal Alcohol and Drug Abuse on the Newborn, edited by Barry Stimmel, MD (AASA 1(3/4), 1982.) *"Authoritative and thought-provoking . . . SHOULD BE CAREFULLY STUDIED BY THOSE RESPONSIBLE FOR THE MANAGEMENT OF DRUG ADDICTION, AND ESPECIALLY BY OBSTETRICIANS AND NEONATAL PEDIATRICIANS." (The British Journal of Psychiatry)*

Recent Advances in the Biology of Alcoholism, edited by Charles S. Lieber, MD, and Barry Stimmel, MD (AASA 1(2), 1982.) *"A VERY VALUABLE HANDBOOK FOR RESEARCHERS AND CLINICIANS interested in alcohol metabolism and its interaction with other drugs, and the endocrine system." (Journal of Studies on Alcohol)*

Opiate Receptors, Neurotransmitters, and Drug Dependence: Basic Science-Clinical Correlates, edited by Barry Stimmel, MD (AASA 1(1), 1981.) *"An exciting, extensive, and innovative approach to the scientific literature in this area." (Journal of Psychoactive Drugs)*

Effects of Substance Abuse Treatment on AIDS Risk Behaviors

Edward Gottheil, MD, PhD
Editor

Barry Stimmel, MD
Series Editor

Effects of Substance Abuse Treatment on AIDS Risk Behaviors has been co-published simultaneously as *Journal of Addictive Diseases*, Volume 17, Number 4 1998.

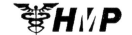

The Haworth Medical Press
An Imprint of
The Haworth Press, Inc.
New York · London

Published by

The Haworth Medical Press, 10 Alice Street, Binghamton, NY 13904-1580 USA

The Haworth Medical Press is an imprint of The Haworth Press, Inc., 10 Alice Street, Binghamton, NY 13904-1580 USA.

Effects of Substance Abuse Treatment on AIDS Risk Behaviors has been co-published simultaneously as *Journal of Addictive Diseases*, Volume 17, Number 4 1998.

The development, preparation, and publication of this work has been undertaken with great care. However, the publisher, employees, editors, and agents of The Haworth Press and all imprints of The Haworth Press, Inc., including The Haworth Medical Press® and Pharmaceutical Products Press®, are not responsible for any errors contained herein or for consequences that may ensue from use of materials or information contained in this work. Opinions expressed by the author(s) are not necessarily those of The Haworth Press, Inc.

Cover design by Thomas J. Mayshock Jr.

Library of Congress Cataloging-in-Publication Data

Effects of substance abuse treatment on AIDS risk behaviors / Edward Gottheil, editor.
    p. cm.
    "Co-published simultaneously as Journal of addictive diseases, vol. 17, no. 4, 1998."
    Includes bibliographical references and index.
    ISBN 0-7890-0696-0 (alk. paper)
    1. AIDS (Disease)–Prevention. 2. Substance abuse–Treatment. 3. AIDS (Disease)–Risk factors. 4 Safe sex in AIDS prevention. 5. Health behavior. I. Gottheil, Edward L. II. Journal of addictive diseases.
RA644.A25E348 1998
616.97'9205–dc21
                                                  98-51374
                                                    CIP

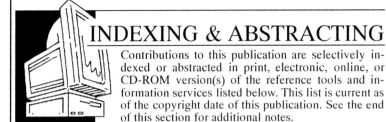

INDEXING & ABSTRACTING

Contributions to this publication are selectively indexed or abstracted in print, electronic, online, or CD-ROM version(s) of the reference tools and information services listed below. This list is current as of the copyright date of this publication. See the end of this section for additional notes.

- *Abstracts in Anthropology*
- *Abstracts of Research in Pastoral Care & Counseling*
- *Academic Abstracts/CD-ROM*
- *ADDICTION ABSTRACTS*
- *ALCONLINE Database*
- *Behavioral Medicine Abstracts*
- *Biosciences Information Service of Biological Abstracts (BIOSIS)*
- *Brown University Digest of Addiction Theory and Application, The (DATA Newsletter)*
- *Cambridge Scientific Abstracts*
- *Child Development Abstracts & Bibliography*
- *CNPIEC Reference Guide: Chinese National Directory of Foreign Periodicals*
- *Criminal Justice Abstracts*
- *Criminal Justice Periodical Index*
- *Criminology, Penology and Police Science Abstracts*
- *Current Contents . . . .* see: *Institute for Scientific Information*
- *Drug Policy Information Clearinghouse*
- *Educational Administration Abstracts (EAA)*
- *EMBASE/Excerpta Medica/Secondary Publishing Division*
- *Family Studies Database (online and CD/ROM)*
- *Health Source: Indexing & Abstracting of 160 selected health related journals, updated monthly*

(continued)

- *Health Source Plus: expanded version of "Health Source" to be released shortly*

- *Index to Periodical Articles Related to Law*

- *Institute for Scientific Information*

- *International Pharmaceutical Abstracts*

- *INTERNET ACCESS (& additional networks) Bulletin Board for Libraries ("BUBL"), coverage of information resources on INTERNET, JANET, and other networks.*

- *Medication Use STudies (MUST) Database*

- *Mental Health Abstracts (online through DIALOG)*

- *NIAAA Alcohol and Alcohol Problems Science Database (ETOH)*

- *PASCAL, c/o Institute de L'Information Scientifique et Technique*

- *Psychological Abstracts (PsycINFO)*

- *Sage Family Studies Abstracts (SFSA)*

- *Sage Urban Studies Abstracts (SUSA)*

- *Social Planning/Policy & Development Abstracts (SOPODA)*

- *Social Work Abstracts*

- *Sociological Abstracts (SA)*

- *SOMED (social medicine) Database*

- *Spanish Technical Information System on Drug Abuse Prevention*

- *Studies on Women Abstracts*

- *Violence and Abuse Abstracts: A Review of Current Literature on Interpersonal Violence (VAA)*

*Special Bibliographic Notes related to special journal issues
(separates) and indexing/abstracting:*

- indexing/abstracting services in this list will also cover material in any "separate" that is co-published simultaneously with Haworth's special thematic journal issue or DocuSerial. Indexing/abstracting usually covers material at the article/chapter level.
- monographic co-editions are intended for either non-subscribers or libraries which intend to purchase a second copy for their circulating collections.
- monographic co-editions are reported to all jobbers/wholesalers/approval plans. The source journal is listed as the "series" to assist the prevention of duplicate purchasing in the same manner utilized for books-in-series.
- to facilitate user/access services all indexing/abstracting services are encouraged to utilize the co-indexing entry note indicated at the bottom of the first page of each article/chapter/contribution.
- this is intended to assist a library user of any reference tool (whether print, electronic, online, or CD-ROM) to locate the monographic version if the library has purchased this version but not a subscription to the source journal.
- individual articles/chapters in any Haworth publication are also available through the Haworth Document Delivery Service (HDDS).

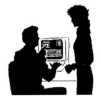

Effects of Substance Abuse Treatment on AIDS Risk Behaviors

CONTENTS

ABOUT THE EDITOR

Edward Gottheil, MD, PhD, is Professor of Psychiatry and Human Behavior at Jefferson Medical College of Thomas Jefferson University in Philadelphia, Pennsylvania, where he is also a research consultant to the division of Alcohol and Drug Abuse Services and an attending psychiatrist. Dr. Gottheil is Associate Editor of *Recent Developments in Alcoholism* and a member of the editorial boards for *The American Journal of Drug and Alcohol Abuse* and *Substance Abuse*. He is Chair of the Biopsychological Research Committee of the American Academy of Psychiatrists in Alcoholism & Addictions and a member of the Board of Directors of the American Academy of Addiction Psychiatry. Dr. Gottheil also serves as principal investigator and co-investigator for several NIDA funded programs. He has co-edited six books and over 140 journal articles on substance abuse, addiction, and treatment.

EDITORIAL

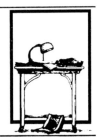

The Problem of HIV/AIDS as Related to Drug Abuse: An Introduction

At the recently held 12th World AIDS conference, some disturbing statistical estimates for 1997 were presented.[1] They included: 30.6 million people infected with HIV worldwide, 5.8 million new cases, and 2.3 million AIDS deaths. At the conference, there was much good news about new findings and advances in treatment, but there was also concern about the need for better preventive measures against the continuing spread of the disease.

Whether substance abuse treatment may serve a preventive function by decreasing HIV-related risk behaviors and thereby reduce the likelihood of developing or transmitting the disease is addressed in the following set of seven papers. These papers were presented at a 1997 ASAM annual confer-

[Haworth co-indexing entry note]: "The Problem of HIV/AIDS as Related to Drug Abuse: An Introduction." Gottheil, Edward. Co-published simultaneously in *Journal of Addictive Diseases* (The Haworth Medical Press, an imprint of The Haworth Press, Inc.) Vol. 17, No. 4, 1998, pp. 1-7; and: *Effects of Substance Abuse Treatment on AIDS Risk Behaviors* (ed: Edward Gottheil, and Barry Stimmel) The Haworth Medical Press, an imprint of The Haworth Press, Inc., 1998, pp. 1-7. Single or multiple copies of this article are available for a fee from The Haworth Document Delivery Service [1-800-342-9678, 9:00 a.m. - 5:00 p.m. (EST). E-mail address: getinfo@haworthpressinc.com].

ence symposium entitled "The Effects of Substance Abuse Treatment on AIDS Risk Behaviors." They include one paper on epidemiology and prevention,[2] one on assessment methodology,[3] and five on treatment and outcome.[4-8] Many of the authors of these papers were Principal Investigators or Co-investigators of a group of R18 developmental grants initiated by NIDA to address the interrelated problems of HIV and drug abuse and much of the data presented came out of the research supported by these grants.

Since transmission occurs by contact with infected body fluids, particularly blood and semen; improved prevention in the absence of an effective vaccine would appear to involve primarily attempts to develop more effective methods for decreasing risky drug and sexual behaviors. Individuals entering substance use treatment programs clearly provide us with opportunities for intervention and prevention. There have been many outcome studies of substance use treatment which have clearly documented that treatment does decrease drug use and that methadone maintenance is particularly effective in reducing injection drug use, thereby directly decreasing at least one form of risky behavior. However, inasmuch as the studies were specially designed to evaluate the effects of drug treatment programs on drug use reduction, scant attention was paid to reductions in other forms of HIV risky behaviors. As a consequence, there is little information in the literature about the effects of substance abuse treatment on AIDS related risk behaviors. Even though most of our drug treatment programs provide their patients with instructional units on HIV/AIDS and its prevention, encourage and make testing available, and offer pre- and post-test counseling, we have not really known to what extent, if any, we are actually changing behaviors and decreasing the likelihood that our patients will contract or spread the disease.

In his paper, Iguchi[4] reported that the risk for HIV transmission among opiate injection drug users (IDUs) was dramatically reduced during a 90-day methadone detoxification program in Baltimore. Along with the expected large decreases that occurred in the number of injection episodes, he described other significant changes in risky behaviors that took place such as where drugs were taken (e.g., shooting galleries) and with whom (e.g., sharing works with multiple strangers). Drug treatment according to Iguchi, then, may reduce HIV transmission risk not only by decreasing the rate and amount of drug use, but also by changing drug taking styles and social behaviors. He suggests that we expand our thinking to include changes in the social environment if we wish to have an impact on risk behaviors and reduce the likelihood of injection related HIV transmission. Changes in social behavior become critically important, of course, in the case of non-injection drug users.

As different from the Northeast, greater proportions of reported AIDS cases in Los Angeles are associated with male-to-male sexual contact and psychostimulant use than with opiate injection drug use. For these populations as well, according to Shoptaw et al.,[5] substance abuse has been shown to be related to high-risk, heterosexual and homosexual HIV-related risk behaviors. While this would seem to suggest that substance use treatment might be beneficial, they note that there have been no previous published reports of non-injection drug treatment as HIV prevention. Similarly, although various psychosocial interventions have been found helpful in treating stimulant abuse, the effects of these treatments on associated HIV risk behaviors have not been assessed. In studies using their Matrix outpatient treatment model, Shoptaw et al. report that while non-injection stimulant users (non-IDUs) were found to engage in high-risk sexual behavior when under the influence, treatment was associated both with decreased drug use and with decreased risky sexual behaviors (e.g., numbers of sexual partners). Moreover, those patients who participated in treatment longer did better. They concluded by emphasizing the usefulness of viewing psychosocial drug treatment as representing a powerful HIV prevention tool for both IDUs and non-IDUs. It would seem to follow then that such programs should be made more available and accessible.

In comparing a Community Reinforcement Approach (CRA) with standard treatment for opioid dependent patients entering a methadone maintenance program, Abbott et al. tested them at intake, and at 6, 12, and 18 months using a battery of instruments which included the Risk for AIDS Behavior (RAB) inventory.[6] As in the previous paper on stimulant users, they also commented about the paucity of published data in regard to whether drug treatment changed HIV behaviors. In their study, they found that for a largely Hispanic group of methadone patients in New Mexico, scores on both the drug use and the sexual behavior subscales of the RAB showed significant improvement at 6, 12, and 18 months when compared with pretreatment levels. The decrease in risky behaviors occurred regardless of whether the patients received standard or CRA treatment. Abbott et al. also conducted careful SCID-P and SCID-II diagnostic evaluations in this study to test the hypotheses that depression and ASPD were associated with increased AIDS risk behaviors. Interestingly, no relationships were found between RAB scores and these or other comorbid psychiatric disorders.

Despite the growing importance of HIV risk assessment for epidemiologic and outcome studies, there are only a limited number of available instruments for this purpose and these, according to Chawarski et al.,[3] have their problems. The questions used by Iguchi[4] and Shoptaw et al.,[5] for example, were selected in accordance with the goals of their particular studies and differed from each other, whereas Abbott et al.[6] employed the more commonly used Risk for AIDS Behavior (RAB) inventory. Clearly, the field would profit greatly if a standardized, reliable, valid and comprehensive instrument were available and used so that findings could be compared across studies. Chawarski et al. discussed the RAB at considerable length in their paper, describing some of its difficulties with respect to psychometric properties, sensitivity, scoring and limited sample of risk exposure categories. Mindful of these shortcomings, they reviewed other instruments and the literature and offered a number of suggestions for an improved and more comprehensive inventory. Following their own advice, they designed and piloted a structured interview that is currently undergoing further modifications. Since the sampling of risks in their interview schedule is rather comprehensive, an interesting feature of their approach is to employ a branching format that permits in-depth questioning of client-specific high-risk behaviors and bypass other non-pertinent areas. Improving our assessment instruments is an ongoing, necessary and challenging task and Chawarski et al. have provided us with some thoughtful observations and suggestions and the promise of an improved instrument. Continued progress will be no less daunting. We will need to learn how to weight and combine items from different domains such as, for example, sexual relations with six different partners in the last month, unprotected sex half of the time, and sharing needles with three individuals on two occasions. To demonstrate validity, we will also have to learn which of our instruments, domains of risk, or items are associated with and predict seroconversion. Perfect measuring sticks in the behavioral field are not easy to come by but advances do seem to be being made.

The RAB was employed by Gottheil et al.[7] in their outcome study of cocaine dependent patients randomly assigned to three months in one of three treatment modalities. It was administered along with a variety of other measures at intake and at 9 month follow-up. Regardless of treatment type, drug use was found to decrease significantly at follow-up as did risky HIV behaviors. In contrast to the findings of Shoptaw et al.,[5] decreased RAB scores were not associated with length of time in treatment. What was found, however, was that ASI drug composite and RAB scores at follow-up were significantly correlated and, more importantly, that decreases in drug use and in risky behaviors from intake to follow-up were also significantly correlated. Patients who reduced their drug intake were those whose risky behaviors decreased. For improvement in HIV-related risk behaviors to occur then, time in treatment may be necessary but not sufficient. In addition to merely attending sessions, more may be required such as participation, involvement, and commitment to day-by-day action during and after the program as witnessed, for example, by decreasing drug use.

Methadone patients who are also abusing cocaine have been found to be engaging in more and higher HIV risk behaviors than those not using cocaine. These are problem patients. Magura et al.[8] compared the needle and risk behaviors for such patients after they had been in treatment for an average of over two years with their risky behaviors prior to entering their large Manhattan methadone maintenance clinic. Heroin use was found to have dropped markedly to an average frequency of about 3 days in the last 30, but cocaine was still being used on about 20 of the last 30 days. Although admitting to their cocaine use, the patients' responses to detailed and specific sets of items showed substantial reductions in both high-risk needle and sexual HIV-related behaviors. The authors observe that many methadone programs discharge patients for continuing cocaine use and they discuss the implications of this issue from different policy perspectives. For example, maintaining these patients in treatment may on the one hand decrease HIV transmission risk, but on the other be disruptive to the promotion of program objectives for recovery from drug addiction. In an interesting methodological maneuver to evaluate the validity of their findings, Magura et al. compared self-reports of heroin use with urinalysis results and redid their analyses excluding those cases in which discrepancies had occurred. The results were nearly identical with no changes in any of the significant findings.

Haverkos[2] discusses the association between HIV/AIDS and drug abuse from an epidemiological perspective focusing on issues as they may relate to prevention. He notes that while the first wave of the HIV/AIDS epidemic, which began in the 1970s and 1980s, involved primarily homosexual men and the second wave which followed shortly thereafter was made up, for the most part, of injection drug users, the third and current wave is more broadly based. The most rapidly increasing rates of AIDS now being reported are among women, minority populations, heterosexual men, and non-injection drug users. While the greatest numbers of cases are still composed of IDUs and men who have sex with men, the continuing and widening spread to other groups through high-risk, HIV-related drug and sexual behaviors is becoming an even more worrisome national public health problem. Regarding prevention, there are no single or simple solutions. However, several prevention strategies have been shown to be helpful in reducing risky behaviors and/or decreasing transmission rates. First and foremost has been drug treatment and especially methadone treatment. A number of community-based outreach interventions have also been useful and have included: education packages, condom and bleach distribution, HIV testing and pre- and post-test counseling, needle and syringe exchanges, and referral to drug treatment and other services. In addition, research on pharmacological and behavioral therapies is receiving support, and several Federal agencies have recently published documents with recommendations favoring treatment and prevention. Nevertheless, despite these positive recommendations, Haverkos points out that little has actually been done to expand treatment slots and services for opiate addicts, and it is estimated that only 15% of injecting opiate users are currently in drug abuse treatment. Cocaine and amphetamine users are also at risk for HIV infection and also have limited access to treatment. He suggests that what is needed are strategies to implement these recommendations to provide more effective and comprehensive prevention and treatment.

The data in our set of papers now provide support for the suggestion made by Haverkos. Would they also justify our asserting that substance abuse treatment is an effective method for HIV risk behavior reduction and transmission prevention? Our authors recommend caution in assuming that any causal connections have been demonstrated since the studies did not involve no-treatment comparison groups and random assignment to treatment or no treatment. In reality, no such studies are possible in an ethical society. Experimental methodology appropriate to physical science disciplines are not always applicable to behavioral investigations[9] or to disciplines such as astronomy where observations, albeit without randomized comparison groups, have yielded reliable information important even to rocket scientists. The findings reported in the present studies were based on more than anecdotes. They were based on the careful and systematic observations of experienced investigators and clinicians in five programs that differed markedly in their methodology and patient samples. For example, sample populations varied from 75% Caucasian to 81% Hispanic and 93% African-American, and sample sizes from 51 to 1415. Three of the programs were located in the Northeast, one in California, and one in New Mexico. One of the programs offered methadone detoxification and one methadone maintenance; one treated cocaine, one stimulants, and one cocaine using methadone patients. All of the programs reported significant decreases in drug use and reductions in HIV-related behaviors; the latter including not only decreases in injection use but also decreases in other risky drug taking behaviors as well as sexual behaviors. There was also evidence that longer treatment times were associated with better outcomes. If not proven according to some standards, there would seem to be a strong presumption that drug treatment works to decrease HIV risky behaviors. For whatever personal or programmatic reasons or causes, drug abusers who receive treatment do better than those who do not both for themselves and for society. Given what we know and what we are learning then, there would seem to be an urgent need to act to make drug treatment more accessible to IDUs and non-IDUs alike in order to decrease drug and sexual risky behaviors and help to reduce the transmission of HIV infection.

Edward Gottheil, MD, PhD

REFERENCES

1. Geneva brings AIDS reality check. Am Med News. July 13, 1998; 41:22-28.

2. Haverkos HW. HIV/AIDS and drug abuse: Epidemiology and prevention. J Addict Dis. 1998; 17(4):91-103.

3. Chawarski MC, Pakes J, Schottenfeld RS. Assessment of HIV risk. J Addict Dis. 1998; 17(4):49-59.

4. Iguchi MY. Drug abuse treatment as HIV prevention: Changes in social drug use patterns might also reduce risk. J Addict Dis. 1998; 17(4):9-18.

5. Shoptaw S, Reback CJ, Frosch DL, Rawson RA. Stimulant abuse treatment as HIV prevention. J Addict Dis. 1998; 17(4):19-32.

6. Abbott PJ, Moore BA, Weller SB, Delaney HD. AIDS risk behavior in opioid dependent patients treated with community reinforcement approach and relationships with psychiatric disorders. J Addict Dis. 1998; 17(4):33-48.

7. Gottheil E, Lundy A, Weinstein SP, Sterling RC. Does intensive outpatient cocaine treatment reduce AIDS risky behaviors? J Addict Dis. 1998; 17(4):61-69.

8. Magura S, Rosenblum A, Rodriguez EM. Changes in HIV risk behaviors among cocaine-using methadone patients. J Addict Dis. 1998; 17(4):71-90.

9. Gottheil E, McLellan AT, Druley KA. Reasonable and unreasonable methodological standards for the evaluation of alcoholism treatment. In: Gottheil E, McLellan AT, Druley KA, eds. Matching patient needs and treatment methods in alcoholism and drug abuse. Springfield, IL: Charles C. Thomas, 1981:371-389.

Drug Abuse Treatment as HIV Prevention: Changes in Social Drug Use Patterns Might Also Reduce Risk

Martin Y. Iguchi, PhD

SUMMARY. Fifty one individuals (37 male and 14 female) were asked to report on the social and behavioral circumstances related to their opiate drug use prior to and during a 90-day methadone detoxification treatment. Data were collected by means of a weekly structured interview. Questions were asked about each occasion of opiate use in the previous week with respect to time, source, cost, social circumstance, etc. Monitored urine samples were tested ×3/week to verify verbal reports. The study demonstrated beneficial effects of the detoxification treatment by showing dramatic decreases in rates and amounts of opiate drug use during treatment. Of perhaps greater significance, large scale changes were also noted in the frequency of use with others. This decline in use with others was most dramatic with respect to strangers and acquaintances. Implications of these observations for HIV transmission are discussed. *[Article copies available for a fee from The Haworth Document Delivery Service: 1-800-342-9678. E-mail address: getinfo@haworthpressinc.com]*

INTRODUCTION

There is little question that drug abuse treatment reduces risk for HIV infection through the straight-forward mechanism of a reduction in frequency

Martin Y. Iguchi, RAND, Drug Policy Research Center, 1700 Main Street, P.O. Box 2138, Santa Monica, CA 90407-2138.

A version of this paper was presented at the American Society for Addiction Medicine Meeting, San Diego, CA, April, 1997.

This research was supported by National Institute on Drug Abuse grants R01 DA06096, DA04104, and T32 DA07209.

[Haworth co-indexing entry note]: "Drug Abuse Treatment as HIV Prevention: Changes in Social Drug Use Patterns Might Also Reduce Risk." Iguchi, Martin Y. Co-published simultaneously in *Journal of Addictive Diseases* (The Haworth Medical Press, an imprint of The Haworth Press, Inc.) Vol. 17, No. 4, 1998, pp. 9-18; and: *Effects of Substance Abuse Treatment on AIDS Risk Behaviors* (ed: Edward Gottheil, and Barry Stimmel) The Haworth Medical Press, an imprint of The Haworth Press, Inc., 1998, pp. 9-18. Single or multiple copies of this article are available for a fee from The Haworth Document Delivery Service [1-800-342-9678, 9:00 a.m. - 5:00 p.m. (EST). E-mail address: getinfo@haworthpressinc.com].

of injection drug use. Maxine Stitzer and I reported, for example, that participants in a 90-day methadone detoxification protocol demonstrated a dramatic decrease in the number of opiate drug use episodes (over 70% was injection drug use) as a result of treatment entry.[1] In that study, opiate use decreased from approximately 13 episodes/week prior to treatment entry down to approximately 2 episodes/week during treatment.

This paper examines additional changes we observed in that study which might also result in a net reduction of risk for HIV transmission. Specifically, I will discuss the impact of treatment on indirect measures of risk for HIV transmission such as where drug use takes place and with whom drug use occurs. The intention is to illustrate how treatment might effect HIV transmission beyond simple reductions in injection frequency.

Where drug use takes place appears to play an important part in drug user's risks for contacting HIV. Numerous studies have reported strong correlations between use of shooting galleries (loosely defined as a place where injection drug users gather to use drugs–and where injection paraphernalia may be rented or otherwise obtained) and HIV infection.[2-5] Latkin et al.[6] also reports that individuals using at injecting friends' residences, shooting galleries, and other semi-public places were significantly more likely to share uncleaned needles.

Who drug users use with is also of obvious importance. I am reporting on self reported use "with" others rather than the more specific "sharing" with others for a number of reasons. First, "needle sharing" is a remarkably imprecise term–especially when considering other related behaviors such as "piggybacking" (drawing drug into a syringe and squirting half the amount into another syringe), "front loading" (removing the needle from the receiving syringe and squirting drug into it), or "backloading" (drawing out the plunger from the receiving syringe and squirting drug into it).[7,8] Second, HIV might also contaminate cookers and spoons used to mix drugs for use, the cotton used to filter the drug solution as it is drawn into the needle, and rinse water which is used to flush needles after use and to prepared drug for injection.[9] Third, many participants stated that they were reluctant to accurately report their needle sharing behavior. Finally, each episode of opiate drug use with another presents a unique opportunity for sharing to occur. As these opportunities accumulate, the likelihood of HIV transmission also increases.

METHODS

Participants

Participants included consecutive new admissions to a 90-day methadone detoxification treatment program at a methadone treatment clinic in Baltimore, MD, USA. Individuals were excluded from the study if they: (1) were older than 55 or younger than 18 years of age; (2) tested positive for pregnancy; or (3) were taking medication by prescription for a physical or psychological disorder. In all, 71 participants (55 men and 16 women) were enrolled in the original research protocol. Of the 71, 20 left treatment within 6 weeks of treatment entry, leaving 51 participants available for this analysis. Table 1 summarizes the standard demographic and background characteristics of the 51 study participants included in this analysis.

General Procedures

The study was approved by the Francis Scott Key Institutional Review Board for human research. More specific details associated with the conduct of this study are reported elsewhere.[1] At the intake appointment, demographic data was collected, study details were read and explained to each participant and informed written consent was obtained. One or two weeks generally

TABLE 1. Demographic and Pre-Treatment Characteristics (N = 51)

	No. (%)	No. (%)	
Gender	37 (73) male	14 (27)	female
Race	13 (25) non-white	38 (75)	white
Marital Status	23 (45) married	28 (55)	single/separated/ divorced
Legal Status	24 (47) free	32 (53)	probation/parole/ trial pending
	Median	Range	
Age (years)	32.0	18-51	
Education (years)	10.0	6-16	
Income Level (dollars/month)	$600	$0-$2400	
Lifetime Duration of Opiate Use (months)	108.0	12-264	

elapsed between intake and treatment admission, depending on receipt of records from other programs or institutions and counselor availability. During this time, participants reported to the clinic once weekly to participate in data collection procedures. After treatment admission, participants were required to report on a daily basis to the clinic where they ingested their methadone dose in a cherry syrup vehicle under nursing supervision. All participants received 40 mg of methadone during an initial three week stabilization period and their dose was then gradually decreased by 4 mg/week over a 10 week period. Medication was delivered in single-blind fashion with patients unaware of their current dose while medication nurses had knowledge of the dosing regimen. Monitored urines were collected from all participants on Monday, Wednesday, and Friday of each week and temperature tested to ensure veracity. Each urine was screened on-site by EMIT® for evidence of opiate, cocaine, or benzodiazepine use. The urine samples were then sent to an independent laboratory for full screen analysis by thin layer chromatography (TLC) which detects use of a wide variety of opiate and non-opiate drugs including morphine, codeine, hydromorphone, propoxyphene, diazepam, oxazepam, barbiturates, phenothiazines, hydroxyzine pamoate (Vistaril®), ethchlorvynol (Placidyl®), and amitriptyline (Elavil®).

The interview process. All interviews were administered by the same research assistant. Participants were interviewed on a weekly basis from the day of intake until treatment termination, using a semi-structured interview. With the exception of the first interview, drug use data was collected with the urinalysis data on-hand so that discrepancies could be immediately noted and probes asked regarding the accuracy of the participant's answers. Inconsistencies between verbal reports and urinalysis results were noted and clarifying probes were asked, particularly when the participant reported no drug use and had submitted a drug-positive sample. Participants were compensated for their time in the amount of $5 per interview.

The first section of the interview asked a series of identical questions about each and every episode of opiate use within the previous week (excluding the interview day) using a brief timeline followback procedure. Participants were asked to carefully review the day and time of each opiate use occasion in the previous week, starting with the previous day and working backwards. If a participant appeared to have difficulty remembering the events of the previous week she was prompted with probes such as, "There was a thunderstorm that day," or "You didn't make it into the clinic that day . . ."

Opiate purchases: source; drug; when; where; and amount obtained. Participants were asked to recall drug purchases for the previous week, to name the specific opiate drug obtained and the amount, to recall dollar cost of the purchase, when purchases were made, and from whom (codenames could be used to identify sources). New drug sources or drug related social contacts were added to a list of different drug sources or drug-related social contacts as they were identified during subsequent interviews.

Opiate use: amount; route; location; and social context. For each drug use occasion, participants were asked to identify the drug used, amount of drug consumed, route of administration, the location of use, the coded identity and social relationship of any individuals using the drug with them, and a question with probes regarding needle sharing.

RESULTS

Impact of Treatment on Frequency of Opiate Use

Figure 1 depicts the total number of opiate use episodes per week reported by the 51 participants included in this analysis for the two week period prior to treatment entry, the two week period immediately following treatment

FIGURE 1. Bar chart comparing the number of self-reported episodes of opiate drug consumption at three different study time points, for the study participants (N = 51) who were in treatment for a minimum of six weeks. The two-week time periods included: (1) baseline–the two-week period just prior to treatment entry; (2) stabilization–weeks one and two of treatment, during which the methadone dose was stabilized at 40 mg; and (3) weeks five and six of treatment.

Average number of opiate use episodes/week (N = 51)

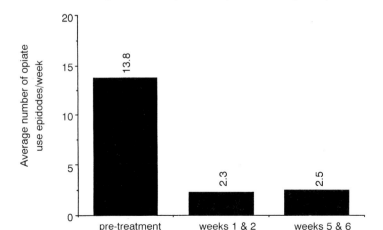

entry, and for weeks 5 and 6 of the 12 week methadone detoxification. The average number of opiate use episodes just prior to treatment entry was 13.8/week (s.d. 9.8; 72% by injection), the average number of opiate use episodes immediately following treatment entry was 2.3/week (s.d. 2.9; 74% by injection), and the average number of opiate use episodes during weeks 5 and 6 was 2.5/week (s.d. 2.8; 56% by injection).

Impact of Treatment on Location of Opiate Use

Subjects reported a significant change in where drugs were used as a result of treatment entry. Prior to treatment entry, nine participants reported using opiates in a shooting gallery. During treatment, no participants reported the use of a shooting gallery during treatment weeks 1 and 2, while only one participant reported the use of a shooting gallery during treatment weeks 5 and 6.

Impact of Treatment on Patterns of Social Drug Use

Treatment also appears to have dramatically altered the social aspect of opiate drug use. Figure 2 depicts changes in the percentage of participants using with acquaintances and strangers, the percentage of participants reporting use with family members or close friends but not with acquaintances or strangers, the percentage of participants reporting that they always used alone during the two week periods, and the percentage of participants reporting that they did not use any opiate drugs during the two week periods. Over one fifth of all participants reported no opiate drug use during the first two weeks and weeks 5 and 6 of treatment. Those reporting that they were always alone when they used opiate drugs increased from 4% to approximately one fifth of all participants. Opiate drug use with acquaintances and strangers declined from 27% of all participants during the pre-treatment period, to 4% of all participants during weeks 5 and 6 of treatment. Opiate drug use with family members and friends declined to a lesser degree, from 69% to approximately half of all participants during treatment.

Impact of Treatment on the Number of Potential HIV Exposures

Figure 3 shows the sum of the number of individuals reported by each study participant as using opiate drugs at the same time and place for each episode of opiate drug use during a given two week period. The data are arranged by relationship to patient (family member/close friend and acquaintance/stranger) and include data from the two weeks prior to treatment entry, treatment weeks 1 and 2, and treatment weeks 5 and 6. In all, the 51 study participants reported more than a thousand potential sharing opportunities

FIGURE 2. The upper left bar chart depicts the percentage of participants reporting opiate drug use with acquaintances and strangers during the two week intervals. The upper right bar chart depicts the percentage of participants reporting opiate drug use with family member and close friends (not including those reporting opiate drug use with acquaintances and strangers), during the two week intervals. The lower left bar chart depicts the percentage of participants reporting that they did not use any opiate drug during the two week intervals. The lower right bar chart depicts the percentage of participants reporting that they were always alone when they used opiate drugs during the two week intervals.

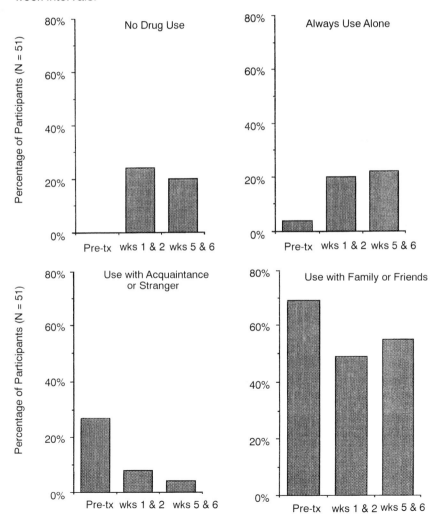

FIGURE 3. Bar chart depicts changes in the sum of the number of individuals reported as also using opiate drugs with the study participant during each occasion of use over three different study time points. Data are reported for use with individuals described as family members or close friends, as well as for those described as acquaintances or strangers.

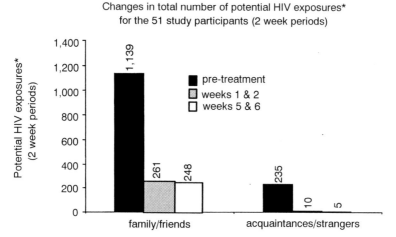

Changes in total number of potential HIV exposures*
for the 51 study participants (2 week periods)

*Defined as the sum of the number of individuals using opiate drugs with the study participant during each occasion of use

(counting each use partner as a separate HIV transmission opportunity) during the 2 weeks prior to treatment entry with family members and friends, as well as the 235 sharing opportunities with acquaintances and strangers. This was reduced during treatment to approximately one fourth the pre-treatment number of potential exposures with family members and friends, and to almost no potential exposures with acquaintances or strangers.

DISCUSSION

As illustrated above, drug abuse treatment may decrease the risk for HIV transmission through a number of mechanisms. First, drug abuse treatment may decrease risk by reducing the number of injection episodes. Second, treatment may decrease injection drug use in higher risk settings such as shooting galleries. Third, treatment may change the social environment in which injections occur–decreasing the use of injectable drugs with others.

Clearly, the reduction in risk for HIV transmission extends well beyond the simple reduction in injection frequency. Indeed, the reduction in risk may extend further. Willems et al.[10] for example, used a snowball sampling procedure to illustrate how primarily dyadic relationships such as those reported above were often just a small portion of larger injection drug using networks. Thus, when an individual breaks off a simple dyadic relationship, they may be isolating themselves from an entire network of risk.

This issue is highlighted by the near elimination of opiate drug use with acquaintances and strangers. Acquaintances and strangers are important as they represent an expansion of the total number of different drug using partners reported by participants, while also representing a "bridge" to other HIV-risk networks. Many participants reported to interviewers that they used with strangers and acquaintances only when they were having difficulty locating drugs, or when they did not have enough money to buy drugs for themselves. Such pressures appear to be a by-product of frequent drug use on a daily basis. It also seems probable that consumption of large quantities of drug also impaired participant judgment, leading to drug use in riskier settings.

This issue of use with family members and close friends is also of great importance. This is true for a number of reasons. First, family members and close friends are identified as co-drug users on a clear majority of occasions. Second, those identifying family members or close friends as co-drug users tended to name the same individuals over and over. Third, close friends and family members might also have multiple other drug use partners–also serving as a potential "bridge" for HIV. Finally, when drug use did occur during treatment, it tended to occur with family members and close friends. This appears to indicate a great need to include couples and family therapy in the treatment process. It suggests a need to expand treatment beyond the individual to these natural drug using groups. Perhaps we should be offering "two for the price of one" treatments or group discounts. Changing social norms is clearly an easier task if the entire peer group can be recruited into treatment.

The data reported above should be interpreted cautiously, however, as we did not have a comparison group for determining how much of the pre- and post-intervention changes were attributable to treatment. Our experience, however, would suggest that the observed changes are unlikely to have occurred in the absence of treatment. Another issue is that the data reported here might not be representative of other treatment modalities and settings. Finally, we do not have data regarding the longer term effects of treatment on these social relationships, and we also know very little about whether the behavior change exhibited by treatment participants alters the social and drug using behaviors of his or her drug using partners.

In summary, the data reported above should be viewed as illustrations of how we might expand our thinking regarding the impact of an intervention on risk behavior. I hope that I have expanded thinking on this issue to include changes in the social environment as it is the constellation of quantitative and qualitative changes which determine the likelihood of injection related HIV transmission.

REFERENCES

1. Iguchi MY, Stitzer ML. Predictors of opiate drug abuse during a 90-day methadone detoxification. Am J Drug Alc Abuse. 1991; 17:279-294.

2. Des Jarlais DC, Friedman SR. Shooting galleries and AIDS: infection probabilities and 'tough' policies. Am J Public Health. 1990; 80:142-144. (Editorial)

3. Marmor M, Des Jarlais DC, Cohen H, et al. Risk factors for infection with human immunodeficiency virus among intraveonous drug abusers in New York City. AIDS. 1987; 1:39-44.

4. Celentano DD, Vlahov D, Cohn S, et al. Risk factors for shooting gallery use and cessation among intravenous drug users. Am J Public Health. 1991; 81:1291-1295.

5. Ouellet LJ, Jimenez AD, Johnson WA, Wiebel WW. Shooting galleries and HIV disease: Variations in places for injecting illicit drugs. Crime and Delinquency. 1991; 37:64-85.

6. Latkin C, Mandell W, Vlahov D, Oziemkowska M, Knowlton A, Celentano, D. My place, your place, and no place: behavior setting as a risk factor for HIV-related injection practices of drug users in Baltimore, Maryland. Am J Community Psych. 1994; 22:415-430.

7. Koester SK, Hoffer L. "Indirect sharing:" Additional HIV risks associated with drug injection. J AIDS Pub Pol. 1994; 9:100-105.

8. Smith AM, Vlahov D, Menon AS, Anthony JC. Terminology for drug injection practices among intravenous drug users in Baltimore. Int J Addict. 1992; 27:435-451.

9. Koester S, Booth R, Wiebel W. The risk of HIV transmission from sharing water, drug-mixing containers and cotton filters among intravenous drug users. Int J Drug Policy. 1990; 1:28-30.

10. Willems J, Iguchi MY, Lidz V, Bux DA. Changes in social networks of injection drug users during methadone maintenance treatment: A study using snowball recruitment and intensive interviews. Subst Use Misuse. 1997; 32:1539-1554.

Stimulant Abuse Treatment as HIV Prevention

Steven Shoptaw, PhD
Cathy J. Reback, PhD
Dominick L. Frosch, BA
Richard A. Rawson, PhD

SUMMARY. Individuals who use illicit stimulants, primarily cocaine and methamphetamine, engage in substantial amounts of HIV-related sexual risk behaviors when under the influence. This paper presents the idea that reductions in stimulant use consequent to drug treatment makes stimulant drug treatment an important HIV prevention tool for

---

Steven Shoptaw is affiliated with Matrix Center, Friends Research Institute, Inc., and West Los Angeles Veterans Administration Medical Center.

Cathy J. Reback is affiliated with Van Ness Recovery House, Prevention Division.

Dominick L. Frosch is affiliated with Matrix Center, and Friends Research Institute, Inc.

Richard A. Rawson is affiliated with Matrix Center, Friends Research Institute, Inc., West Los Angeles Veterans Administration Medical Center, and UCLA School of Psychiatry and Biobehavioral Sciences.

Address correspondence to: Richard A. Rawson, PhD, Matrix Center, 10350 Santa Monica Boulevard, Suite 330, Los Angeles, CA 90025.

The authors gratefully acknowledge support from Contract Number H204213 from the U.S. Centers for Disease Control and Prevention and the County of Los Angeles, Department of Health Services, Office of AIDS Programs and Policy for Dr. Reback's street outreach study. Dr. Shoptaw's contribution to this work was supported by NIDA grant R44 DA08786. The authors also want to recognize the generous and consistent support provided by Friends Medical Science Research Center, Inc., for their grants administration and administrative support.

[Haworth co-indexing entry note]: "Stimulant Abuse Treatment as HIV Prevention." Shoptaw, Steven et al. Co-published simultaneously in *Journal of Addictive Diseases* (The Haworth Medical Press, an imprint of The Haworth Press, Inc.) Vol. 17, No. 4, 1998, pp. 19-32; and: *Effects of Substance Abuse Treatment on AIDS Risk Behaviors* (ed: Edward Gottheil, and Barry Stimmel) The Haworth Medical Press, an imprint of The Haworth Press, Inc., 1998, pp. 19-32. Single or multiple copies of this article are available for a fee from The Haworth Document Delivery Service [1-800-342-9678, 9:00 a.m. - 5:00 p.m. (EST). E-mail address: getinfo@haworthpressinc.com].

19

this high-risk population. Data are presented to describe many of the HIV-related sexual risks reported by out-of-treatment methamphetamine users and by cocaine and methamphetamine abusers at treatment entry and six months post treatment entry. Overall, our findings demonstrate that following initiation of a treatment episode, stimulant abusers demonstrate significant and relevant reductions in HIV-related sexual behaviors, primarily by reducing the number of sexual partners. Reasons for why stimulant treatment corresponds to HIV transmission risk reductions and suggestions for implementing prevention messages in treatment settings are offered. *[Article copies available for a fee from The Haworth Document Delivery Service: 1-800-342-9678. E-mail address: getinfo@haworthpressinc.com]*

INTRODUCTION

The vast majority of Americans with HIV contracted the virus by engaging in one or more drug use or sexual behaviors that resulted in sharing blood or semen containing the virus. The primary method for controlling the spread of HIV continues to be interventions that promote adopting safer sexual and drug use behaviors among individuals in high-risk groups (i.e., men who have sex with men–MSM and/or injection drug users–IDUs) and non-injection drugs that promote high-risk sexual behaviors such as methamphetamine use among gay and bisexual males. Many prevention interventions are conducted in contexts in which HIV-related sexual risk behaviors are likely to occur (e.g., sex clubs, bathhouses, parks) or in situations in which drug users might be influenced to change specific drug use behaviors (e.g., at needle exchanges, in methadone clinics, on the streets).

Interventions designed to change HIV-related sexual behaviors, particularly among gay and bisexual men have showed remarkable effects in getting individuals to adopt safer sexual behaviors,[1] even if only in the short run.[2] Prevention interventions designed for MSMs have slowed the rate of HIV spread, especially among older urban males.[3] Yet, substantial proportion of younger urban males continue to report engaging in AIDS-related sexual risk behaviors, with corresponding levels of HIV-seroconversion being observed.[3,4] Proportional increases in nationwide reported AIDS cases among African Americans, Latinos, women, and youth[5] indicate that successful sexual behavior change programs have yet to be implemented for individuals in these communities.

Drug use behaviors are shown to be more amenable to change than sexual behaviors.[6] IDUs have a good general knowledge of how to clean needles prior to injection,[7] though education programs to instruct on needle cleaning practices have demonstrated increases in technical proficiency[8] and reductions in reported needle sharing behaviors.[9,10] More recently the best recommendation for stopping injection related HIV transmission among IDUs is for accessibility to needle exchange[11] and many readily avail themselves of needle exchange. However, several research groups have documented significantly increased risks for HIV infection additional to injection risks among opiate dependent individuals who use cocaine,[12,13] risks that may even exceed those due to needle use.

Non-injection drug use, particularly of psychostimulants, carries with it substantial risks for HIV transmission. In a landmark study, Edlin and colleagues[14] demonstrated that urban crack cocaine smokers reportedly engaged in alarming rates of HIV-related sexual risk behaviors associated with their drug use and concluded that crack use promotes heterosexual transmission of HIV. Wambach and colleagues documented a similar association for female crack smokers.[15] Khalsa and colleagues[16] reviewed the literature and concluded that HIV-related risks consequent to crack cocaine use can arise from semen exchange during frequent sexual episodes without condom usage, blood-to-blood contact from open sores due to hot crack pipes, and penile and vaginal abrasions that can occur from sexual episodes prolonged due to delayed orgasms. These types of risks are clearly additive and independent to those associated with injection drug behaviors.

Among gay and bisexual men, stimulant use has long been associated with HIV-related sexual risk behaviors. Stall and colleagues[17] initially noted that the number of drugs reported used predicted high-risk sexual behavior in a stepwise fashion. Associations between substance use and HIV-related sexual risk behaviors among gay and bisexual men have been documented by many groups.[18-30] Particular associations have been reported between unprotected anal intercourse with the use of amphetamines and "poppers," both of which are used to enhance the sexual experience.[19,20,23,25-27,30]

Substance Abuse Treatment as HIV Prevention

The correspondence between illicit drug use and HIV-related risk behaviors is well established and has prompted some to suggest that the treatment of substance abuse disorders may have a significant impact as an HIV prevention method. Evaluating the preventive value of narcotic treatment programs, Moss and colleagues[31] followed 3,000 in- and out-of-treatment opiate users in San Francisco and concluded that stable methadone maintenance is the most protective behavior against HIV-seroconversion in this high risk group. Documenting whether HIV risk reduction might result from substance abuse treatment for non-injection drug users, primarily stimulant users, is complicated by individual variation of sexual risk behaviors that often depend upon factors such as the users' sexual orientation (e.g., homosexual, bisexual, or heterosexual), relationship with other individuals at high risk for

HIV infection (e.g., wife of a bisexual drug user), and social class (e.g., housed middle class user or homeless sex worker).

There are no published reports of non-injection substance abuse treatment as HIV prevention. However, there is evidence that HIV-prevention programs in non-injection drug treatment settings can be effective in reducing HIV risk behaviors. Malow and Ireland[32] reported that among 111 males, mostly heterosexual veteran inpatients treated for cocaine dependence, AIDS-risk knowledge increased with intervention, while reported condom use was low at baseline and continued low throughout.

The current paper provides a report on our group's work to evaluate the HIV-related risk behaviors for non-injecting stimulant users seeking treatment in Los Angeles. The report includes data from three different studies which investigated the relationship between stimulant (cocaine and methamphetamine) use and HIV risk behaviors. Particular attention is focused on associations between treatment outcome and subsequent reported HIV-related sexual risk behaviors.

Community-Based Intervention to Non-Treatment Seeking Drug Users

In Los Angeles, 80% of reported AIDS cases (26,381/33,130) are due to male-to-male sexual contact[33] and an additional 7% of cases are due to injection drug use combined with the MSM classification. Hence, in 87% of AIDS cases in Los Angeles County, male-to-male sexual contact was *the* factor, or *one of the two* risk factors, associated with HIV transmission. These numbers clearly illustrate the importance of intervening with these groups in Los Angeles considering the overwhelming involvement of individuals from these groups in HIV transmission. An understanding of factors that influence risk-taking behaviors, both when under and when not under the influence of illicit drugs in this MSM group has substantial importance concerning HIV transmission in Los Angeles.

The use of methamphetamine has been documented to be an important element integrated into the sexual behaviors of many MSMs in Western cities in the United States. In Los Angeles County, the city of Hollywood is the "skid row," for the gay drug using communities. The street life in Hollywood is very similar to that of Downtown Los Angeles, with the exception that it is primarily gay. Injection drug equipment is shared both on the streets and in shooting galleries, sex is exchanged for money and/or drugs, and many are homeless or living collectively in inexpensive hotels.

In response to the needs of this extremely high-risk population, the Prevention Division of the Van Ness Recovery House designed and implemented a street-based HIV education and prevention program targeting gay, bisexual, lesbian, and transgender (male-to-female) drug users in Hollywood. The intervention is based on a harm reduction model, measuring outcome as any social, psychological, or physical reduction in the harm that results from drug use. All HIV interventions took place where high-risk sex and/or drug-related activities occur such as street corners, bus stops, parking lots, parks, cruising areas, bars, bathhouses, sex clubs, abandoned buildings, hotels, coffee houses, fast food stands, and mini markets.

The intervention model was developed to provide services to a street-based population, many of whom are homeless. Services are provided by indigenous community outreach workers. Upon contact, gifts such as hygiene kits, are given to establish trust and aid with immediate needs. Interventions include peer-to-peer counseling, education/support groups on topics such as addiction, sexuality and homophobia, and staying safe. All participants are offered condoms, bleach kits, and other risk reduction supplies. After trust is established, outreach workers conduct a brief HIV risk and needs assessment which includes questions regarding their substance use, sexual behaviors, and high risk activities. Direct linked referrals that assist with immediate and long-term needs are provided following the risk assessment.

Findings: A total of 1,415 individuals participated in this survey, 1,092 (77.2%) reported their sexual identification as gay or bisexual males. Supporting earlier reports,[21,34] MSM participants reported widespread use of methamphetamine within this urban West Coast group. Almost one-half (48%) of the sample of 1,092 MSMs reported having used methamphetamine in the previous 30 days. Methamphetamine was the third most frequently used substance following alcohol and marijuana. The association between methamphetamine use and HIV-related drug use and sexual risk behaviors are evident from Table 1. Among MSM injection drug users in this sample, 87% reported methamphetamine use in the previous 30 days, which is a rate higher than for any other drug. In addition, sharing needles (54%) and trading sex for drugs (74%) further increased the HIV transmission risk for this group. Even methamphetamine users who are noninjectors reported a significant amount of HIV-related sexual behaviors as indicated by the high rate of sex for trade behavior (58%).

These data and others reported by this group[21] establish that methamphetamine use is associated with very high rates of HIV risk behavior by some gay and bisexual males. The categories of risk behaviors include injection drug use, needle sharing, involvement in selling/trading sex for money and drugs, and high risk sex without trade particularly in sexually charged arenas such as gay bathhouses and sex clubs. Of special importance with this group is the association of methamphetamine use with reported high-risk sexual behavior.[21] It seems reasonable that one method for slowing the rate of

TABLE 1. Frequencies of HIV-Risk Behaviors Among Gay and Bisexual Male (MSM)

Number of MSM in survey–1092	n	%
Number/Percent of MSM using MA during previous 30 days	524	48%
Number/Percent of MSM who inject drugs (IDU)	222	20.3%
Of the MSM, IDU (n = 222), number/percent who use MA in last 30 days	192	87%
Of the MSM, IDU, MA Users (n = 192), number/percent who share needles	104	54%
Of the MSM, IDU, MA Users (n = 192), number/percent who provide sex for money or drugs	142	74%
Of the MSM, non-IDU, MA Users (n = 199), number/percent who provide sex for money or drugs	115	58%

HIV-transmission in this extremely high-risk group is to develop successful strategies for reducing the use of stimulants, especially methamphetamine.

Treatment of Stimulant Abusers as HIV Risk Reduction

The evidence demonstrating the interconnectedness of stimulant use and elevated reported rates of HIV risk behaviors suggests that successful treatments for stimulant abuse disorders may hold promise as useful strategies for HIV risk reduction. Currently, there are no medication treatments for stimulant dependence with demonstrated efficacy.[35] Non-pharmacologic treatments including the community reinforcement approach[36] and relapse prevention[37] have been reported to have considerable empirical support as stimulant abuse treatments. However, the impact of these psychosocial interventions on associated HIV risk behaviors have not been assessed.

Another psychosocial approach for stimulant abuse treatment which has evidence of clinical value is the Matrix model.[38-40] This model of stimulant abuse treatment has been shown to be associated with reduced cocaine use, improvements in substance use related problems as measured by the Addiction Severity Index, and improvements in a range of other measures of functioning as measured by the Basis-32.[41] The clinical impact of this treatment approach has been found to produce a comparable treatment response for cocaine and methamphetamine users.[42] A detailed description of the approach has been previously published[39] and the Matrix Manual for Stimulant Abuse Treatment has been published for dissemination.[43]

There have been a number of demonstrations which support the value of this stimulant abuse treatment approach in reducing HIV risk behavior. As part of a NIDA-funded demonstration project (Stimulant Abuse Treatment to Reduce the Spread of HIV, Richard Rawson, PI 1989-1994, R18 DA06185), HIV risk behaviors were assessed using the NIDA/WAVE[44] instrument before and after stimulant abusers were entered into the 6 months treatment experience of the Matrix protocol. Results from this study supported the usefulness of this approach as a method for reducing both the use of stimulants as well as for reducing the associated HIV risk behaviors.

A total of 290 stimulant abusers (232 cocaine, 58 methamphetamine) were admitted to the demonstration project and participated in the outpatient program for up to 6 months. Figure 1 illustrates the association of treatment participation in the Matrix treatment elements with a reduction in the number of sexual partners. The number of sexual partners reported by subjects during the 6 months period before treatment was significantly reduced at the 6 month post admission follow-up point. This reduction was significant for

FIGURE 1. Reduction in sexual partners by sexual orientation.

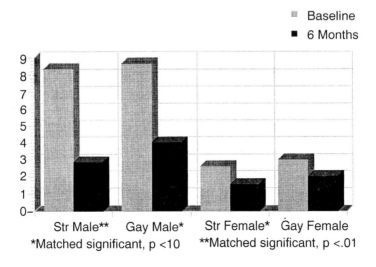

Str Male**   Gay Male*   Str Female*   Gay Female
*Matched significant, p <10   **Matched significant, p <.01

FIGURE 2. Changes in safe sex by treatment variables.

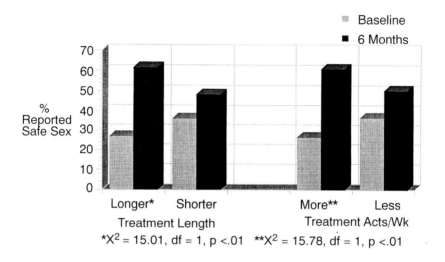

*X² = 15.01, df = 1, p <.01   **X² = 15.78, df = 1, p <.01

heterosexual males (p < .01), and approached significance for gay and bi-sexual males and heterosexual females (0. 1 > p > .05).

Figure 2 illustrates the relationship between an improvements in a "safer sex" composite measure and treatment "dose." Subjects who participated in longer treatment episodes (more than 20 weeks) and in a higher frequency of treatment activities during treatment (more than 2 for week) reported significantly increased safe sex composite scores. Those who had shorter and less intensive "doses" in the psychosocial protocol did not demonstrate statistically significant increases in the safe sex measure.

These data indicating a relationship between treatment in the Matrix outpatient protocol and reported reductions in HIV risk behavior have been further demonstrated in a report by Shoptaw and colleagues.[45] In this report, 157 of the cocaine abusing subjects in the demonstration project provided data from the NIDA/WAVE questionnaire at baseline and at 6 months follow-up evaluations. Subjects were dichotomized into those who were engaging in "safer sex" and those not engaging in "safer sex" according to the following criteria. Safer sex was defined as: (1) serial monogamy for the 6 months preceding the interview, or (2) for those with multiple partners, condom use at each sexual encounter, and (3) no exchanges of sex for drugs or cash, and (4) no sexual intercourse under the influence of drugs and alcohol.

Using this definition of safer sex, 35% of the study sample (n = 55/157) met criteria for "safer sex" at baseline prior to treatment entry. At the 6

TABLE 2. Specific Sexual Behavior Changes over 6 Months (N = 157)

	Baseline	6 Months			
	M	M	F	p	
Condom use	2.29	2.10	3.01	ns	
# of reported sex partners	5.32	2.47	36.32	.001	
Sex under the influence of drugs	2.49	1.64	61.22	.001	
Sex under the influence of alcohol	2.05	1.50	33.50	.001	
	M	M	X^2	OR	p
Drugs for sex	32.9%	14.8%	23.04	10.09	.001
Cash for sex	28.1%	10.3%	5.28	3.39	.05

month post admission follow-up point, 69% (n = 109) of subjects met criteria for "safer sex." This increase in the safer sex percentage was statistically significant X^2 (1,157) = 21.25, p < .001). Table 2 lists the changes in specific risk behaviors from baseline to 6 months. As shown in the Table, participation in treatment with the 6 month Matrix outpatient approach was associated with a significant improvement in all categories of risky behavior measured, except for condom use. Additional details on the relationship between treatment and reduced HIV risk behavior use are included in Shoptaw et al., in press.

DISCUSSION

Our findings document that non-injection stimulant users engage in high rates of HIV-related sexual behaviors when under the influence. Our data also indicate that when given access to stimulant drug treatment, stimulant users significantly and substantially reduce the extent they engage in HIV-related sexual risk behaviors. However, our findings do not provide for a prospective test of the value of stimulant drug treatment as HIV prevention. Rather, these findings strongly indicate that reductions in stimulant use that correspond with treatment allow individuals to make more thoughtful decisions regarding their sexual behavior. Corresponding reductions in HIV transmission in these high risk groups would reasonably follow. In such manner, stimulant drug treatment, in itself represents a potentially powerful HIV prevention method.

Our data and the relevant literature are also consistent in indicating that substance abuse treatment settings are vital delivery points for HIV prevention messages intended for drug abusers. To this point, prevention messages for drug abusers have focused on modifying injection behaviors, largely due to the high seroprevalence of HIV among IDUs along the East Coast.[46] Yet in areas of the country that have stable, low rates of HIV among IDUs, such as urban areas in the Western United States, non-injection stimulants represent a class of drugs whose use is associated with substantially greater risks for facilitating HIV transmission than injectable drugs (i.e., heroin). Unfortunately, the literature evaluating current prevention interventions suggests that sexual risk behaviors consequent to non-injection stimulant use are difficult to modify, especially over long periods. Given this understanding, it is prudent to consider stimulant use as a marker for potential HIV exposure among all such treatment seeking individuals. Further, it is crucial that drug abuse clinicians and researchers better understand the ways in which drug abusers engage in high-risk behaviors while under the influence of these powerful drugs as an initial step to developing effective HIV prevention messages.

Better understandings of the correspondences between stimulant use and sexual behaviors will facilitate design of HIV prevention interventions that can be successfully implemented into stimulant treatment programs. For example, several studies have replicated the finding that overall, individuals fail to increase condom use following prevention programs.[2,10] However, more careful studies of sexual behavior have demonstrated that individuals in high risk groups report they are able to implement condom use with anonymous partners or when being paid for sex.[7,15,47] Preliminary clinical findings from Dr. Reback's street outreach data indicate that even individuals in the highest risk groups for HIV transmission–gay male, methamphetamine using, sex workers–implement condom use during sex work following brief prevention interventions. Such findings give hope since these are the contexts and the individuals that carry the highest risks for HIV transmission. When relevant prevention information is presented in such manner, individuals perceive the increased risks and modify their behavior when in those contexts. This targeted, highly specific approach allows treatment professionals to set behavioral goals that clients can attain and recognizes that few individuals will use or need to use condoms during 100% of their sexual experiences.

Research demonstrating the preventive value of drug treatment as HIV prevention presents a variety of difficult methodological issues. Unlike the more monolithic group of IDUs (e.g., opiate injectors), who engage in identical behaviors that present risk for exposure to a variety of infectious agents including HIV, non-injection stimulant users differ to the extent and type of sexual risk behaviors they engage that correspond with their drug use. This presents tricky ethical and reality-based problems for carefully evaluating drug use and sexual behavior correspondences among non-injection, stimulant users.[48] Both drug use and sexual behavior are private events and researchers must rely on retrospection, which introduces a host of biases as a measurement technique. Drug use and sexual behavior also both invoke strong feelings of pleasure and to the extent that drug use and sexual behavior become conditioned together, it can be especially difficult to untangle factors that relate to drug relapse and those that relate to impulsive sexual behavior. Further, researchers have documented that drug treatment can change subsequent levels of reported HIV-related sexual risk behaviors, though it is remains unexamined whether effective sexual risk reduction interventions lead to corresponding changes in drug use behavior.

A related methodological difficulty is that most drug users risks for HIV exposure vary depending upon their current drug use status. Drug dependence is a chronic, relapsing condition and few stimulant abusers adopt a lifestyle of abstinence consequent to a single drug treatment episode. During periods of abstinence, risks for HIV exposure may be relatively slim, primarily due to improved decision making. Individuals are substantially more likely to engage in behaviors that place them at risk for HIV transmission when under the influence of stimulants.[21] Stimulant abusers also experience differing risks for HIV exposure. Female cocaine smokers in rural areas may be dramatically less likely to encounter HIV than when male methamphetamine users who have sex with other men. Despite these risk differences, providing access to treatment during the active phase of a substance abuse disorder may limit harm to public health and decrease of spread in the population.

The treatment setting offers an excellent opportunity for addressing sexual behavior relative to drug use since individuals in treatment clients are often more open to considering behavior changes. Counselors make excellent agents for delivering prevention messages due to the trust often yielded them by clients. Yet a challenge exists for the treatment field since the prevention data indicate that adopting absolutist interventions regarding sexual behavior does not result in behavior change with these high-risk populations. Holding to the idea that all should use condoms all the time fails to equip individuals with a range of response options for high-risk situations, i.e., when under the influence or when in highly charged sexual contexts. One important avenue of investigation is to evaluate whether there are HIV-related sexual risk behavior reductions that individuals can accomplish–even when under the influence of stimulants. These interventions might include such basic suggestions as reducing a stimulant binge by one day, using condoms when having sex with unknown partners, or having oral instead of anal or vaginal sex. Though these interventions clearly confront drug treatment professionals' adherence to abstinence-based models, implementation of such may provide their drug-using clients with the skills to avoid exposure to HIV.

REFERENCES

1. Kelly JA. Changing HIV Risk Behavior: Practical Strategies. New York: The Guilford Press, 1995.

2. Stall R, Ekstrand M, Pollack L, McKusick L, Coates TJ. Relapse from safer sex: the next challenge for AIDS prevention efforts. J Acquir Immune Defic Syndr. 1990; 3:1181-1187.

3. Holmberg SD. Emerging epidemiologic patterns of HIV in the United States. AIDS Res Hum Retroviruses. 1994; 10:56.

4. Dean L, Meyer IH. HIV prevention and sex behavior in a cohort of young New York gay men (aged 18-24). J AIDS Hum Retrovirology. 1995; 8(2):208-211.

5. Centers for Disease Control and Prevention. HIV/AIDS Surveillance Report. 1996; 8(2): 5-6.

6. Baker A, Heather N, Wodak A, Dixon J, Holt P. Evaluation of a cognitive-behavioural intervention for HIV prevention among injecting drug users. AIDS. 1993; 7:247-256.

7. Liebman I, Mulia N, McIlvaine D. Risk behavior for HIV infection of intravenous drug users and their sexual partners recruited from street settings in Philadelphia. J Drug Issues. 1992; 22(4):867-884.

8. Saxon AJ, Calsyn DA. Comparison of HIV-associated risk behaviors of primary intravenous stimulant users and opioid-addicted subjects on methadone maintenance. Am J Addict. 1992; 1(4):304-314.

9. Boatler JF, Knight K, Simpson DD. Assessment of an AIDS intervention program during drug abuse treatment. J Subst Abuse Treat. 1994; 11(4):367-372.

10. Dengelegi L, Weber J, Torquato S. Drug users' AIDS-related knowledge, attitudes, and behaviors before and after AIDS education sessions. Public Health Rep. 1990; 105(5):504-510.

11. Jones TS, Wright-DeAgilero L, Miles J. Sterile injection: The "gold standard" for drug users who continue to inject. Paper presented at the 1995 NIDA Conf. on AIDS and Drug Abuse. June 9-10, 1995, Scottsdale, AZ.

12. Cohen E, Navaline H, Metzger D. High-risk behaviors for HIV: a comparison between crack-abusing and opioid-abusing African-American women. J Psychoactive Drugs. 1994; 26(3):233-241.

13. Grella CE, Anglin MD, Wugalter SE. Cocaine and crack use and HIV risk behaviors among high-risk methadone maintenance clients. Drug Alcohol Depend. 1995; 37:15-21.

14. Edlin BR, Irwin KL, Faruque S, McCoy CB, Word C, Serrano Y, Inciardi JA, Bowser BP, Schilling RF, Holmberg SD, Multicenter Crack Cocaine and HIV Infection Study Team. Intersecting epidemics–crack cocaine use and HIV infection among inner-city young adults. N Engl J Med. 1994; 331:1422-7.

15. Wambach KG, Byers JB, Harrison DF, Levine P, Imershein AW, Quadagno DM, Maddox K. Substance use among women at risk for HIV infection. J Drug Educ. 1992; 22(2):131-146.

16. Khalsa ME, Kowalewski MR, Lunn R, Anglin MD, Miller HA. AIDS-related knowledge, beliefs and risk behaviors in a sample of crack addicts. J Drug Issues. 1994; 24(3):537-553.

17. Stall R, McKusick L, Wiley J, Coates TJ, Ostrow DG. Alcohol and drug use during sexual activity and compliance with safe sex guidelines for AIDS: the AIDS behavioral research project. Health Educ Q. 1986; 13(4):359-371.

18. Barrett DC, Bolan G, Joy D, Counts Doll L, Harrison J. Coping strategies, substance use, sexual activity, and HIV sexual risks in a sample of gay male STD patients. J Appl Soc Psychol. 1995; 25(12): 1058-1072.

19. Burchman J, Tindall B, Marmor M, Cooper D, Berry G, Penny R. Incidence and risk factors for human immunodeficiency virus seroconversion in a cohort of Sydney homosexual men. Med J Aust. 1989; 150:634-639.

20. de Wit JBF, van Griensven JP. Time from safer to unsafe sexual behaviour among homosexual men. AIDS. 1994; 8:123-126.

21. Frosch D, Shoptaw S, Huber A, Rawson RA, Ling W. Sexual HIV risk among gay and bisexual male methamphetamine abusers. J Subst Abuse Treat. (in press).

22. McCusker J, Westenhouse J, Stoddard AM, Zapka JG, Zorn MW, Mayer KH. Use of drugs and alcohol by homosexually active men in relation to sexual practices. J Acquir Immune Defic Syndr. 1990; 3:729-736.

23. Messiah A, Bucquet D, Mettetal JF, Larroque B, Rouzioux C, the Alain Brugeat Physician Group. Factors correlated with homosexually acquired human Immunodeficiency virus infection in the era of "safer sex": was the prevention message clear and well understood? Sex Transm Dis. 1993; 20(1):51-58.

24. Mulry G, Kalichman SC, Kelly JA. Substance use and unsafe sex among gay men: global versus situational use of substances. J Sex Educ Ther. 1994; 20(3): 175-184.

25. Myers T, Rowe CJ, Tudiver FG, Hurts RG, Jackson EA, Orr KW, Bullock SL. HIV, substance use and related behaviour of gay and bisexual men: an examination of the talking sex project cohort. Br J Addiction. 1992; 87:207-214.

26. Paul JP, Stall RD, Crosby M, Barrett DC, Midanik LT. Correlates of sexual risk-taking among gay male substance abusers. Addiction. 1994; 89:971-983.

27. Paul JP, Stall R, Davis F. Sexual risk for HIV transmission among gay/bisexual men in substance-abuse treatment. AIDS Educ Prev. 1993; 5(1):11-24.

28. Reback CJ. The social construction of a gay drug: Methamphetamine use among gay and bisexual males in Los Angeles. Technical report funded by contract #93427 from the City of Los Angeles, AIDS Coordinator, 1997.

29. Silvestre Al, Lyter DW, Valdiserri RO, Huggins J, Rinaldo CR, Jr. Factors related to seroconversion among homo- and bisexual men after attending a risk-reduction educational session. AIDS. 1989; 3:647-650.

30. Stall R, Wiley J. A comparison of alcohol and drug use patterns of homosexual and heterosexual men: the San Francisco men's health study. Drug Alcohol Depend. 1988; 22:63-73.

31. Moss AR, Vranizan K, Gorter R, Bacchetti P, Watters J, Osmond D. HIV seroconversion in intravenous drug users in San Francisco, 1985-1990. AIDS. 1994; 8:223-231.

32. Malow RM, Ireland SJ. HIV risk correlates among non-injection cocaine dependent men in treatment. AIDS Educ Prev. 1996; 8(3):226-235.

33. HIV Epidemiology Program, Los Angeles County Department of Health Services. Advanced HIV Disease (AIDS) Surveillance Summary. April 15, 1997; 1-23.

34. Gorman EM, Morgan P, Lambert EY. Qualitative research considerations and other issues in the study of methamphetamine use among men who have sex with other men. NIDA Res Monogr. 1995; 157:156-181.

35. Meyers RE. New pharmacotherapies for cocaine dependence revisited. Arch Gen Psychiatry. 1992; 49(11):900-904.

36. Higgins ST, Budney AJ, Bickel WK, Badger GJ, Foerg FE, Ogden D. Outpatient behavioral treatment for cocaine dependence: one-year outcome. Exp Clin Psychopharmacol. 1995; 3(2):205-212.

37. Carroll KM, Rounsaville BJ, Niche C, Gordon LT, Wirtz PW, Gavin F. One-year follow-up of psychotherapy and pharmacotherapy for cocaine dependents. Arch Gen Psychiatry. 1994; 51:989-997.

38. Rawson RA, Obert JL, McCann MJ, Mann AJ. Cocaine treatment outcome: Cocaine use following inpatient, outpatient, and no treatment. Proceedings of the Committee on Problems of Drug Dependence. NIDA Res Monogr. 1985; 67:271-277.

39. Rawson RA, Shoptaw SJ, Obert JL, McCann MJ, Hasson AL, Marinelli-Casey PJ, Brethen PR, Ling W. An intensive outpatient approach for cocaine abuse treatment: the Matrix model. J Subst Abuse Treat. 1995; 12(2):117-127.

40. Shoptaw S, Rawson RA, McCann MJ, Obert IL. The Matrix model of outpatient stimulant abuse treatment: Evidence of efficacy. J Addict Dis. 1994; 13(4):25-34.

41. Zogg J, McCann MJ, Rawson RA, Ling W. Substance abuse treatment outcomes in a private program. Presented at the American Society of Addiction Medicine Conference, San Diego, California, April 1997.

42. Huber A, Ling W, Shoptaw S, Gulati V, Brethen P, Rawson R. Integrating treatments for methamphetamine abuse: a psychosocial perspective. J Addict Dis. 1997; 16(4):41-50.

43. Rawson RA, Obert JL, McCann MJ, Smith DP, Scheffey EH. The Neurobehavioral Treatment Manual. Beverly Hills, CA: The Matrix Center, 1989.

44. Longshore D, Hsieh S, Anglin MD. AIDS knowledge and attitudes among injection drug users: The issue of reliability. AIDS Educ Prev. 1992; 4(1):29-40.

45. Shoptaw S, Frosch D, Rawson RA, Ling W. Cocaine abuse counseling as HIV prevention. AIDS Educ Prev. 1997; 9(3):15-24.

46. Steel E, Haverkos HW. Epidemiologic studies of HIV/AIDS and Drug Abuse. A J Drug Alcohol Abuse. 1992; 18(2):167-175.

47. Anderson JE, Cheney R, Clatts M, Faruque S, Kipke M, Long A, Mills S, Toomey K, Wiebel W. HIV risk behavior, street outreach, and condom use in eight high-risk populations. AIDS Educ Prev. 1996; 8(3):191-204.

48. Leigh BC, Stall R. Substance use and risky sexual behavior for exposure to HIV. Am Psychol. 1993; 48(10):1035-1045.

AIDS Risk Behavior
in Opioid Dependent Patients Treated
with Community Reinforcement Approach
and Relationships
with Psychiatric Disorders

Patrick J. Abbott, MD
Brent A. Moore, MS
Susan B. Weller, MS
Harold D. Delaney, PhD

SUMMARY. This study examined the Community Reinforcement Approach's (CRA) effect on AIDS risk behaviors and the relationship

Patrick J. Abbott is Medical Director, Treatment Division, Center on Alcoholism, Substance Abuse, and Addictions (CASAA) and Assistant Professor of Psychiatry, University of New Mexico, School of Medicine, 2350 Alamo SE, Albuquerque, NM 87106.

Brent A. Moore is Statistician, Research Data Services, Center on Alcoholism, Substance Abuse, and Addictions (CASAA) and a PhD candidate in Psychology, University of New Mexico. He is now at the Center for Studies on Alcohol, at Westat, Rockville, MD.

Susan B. Weller is Project Director of NIDA funded research project "Community Reinforcement/Relapse Prevention Approaches to Treating Heroin Abuse," Treatment Division, Center on Alcoholism, Substance Abuse, and Addictions (CASAA), University of New Mexico Mental Health Programs.

Harold D. Delaney is Professor of Psychology, University of New Mexico.

Address correspondence to: Patrick J. Abbott at the above address.

This research was supported by a grant from the National Institute on Drug Abuse (5 R18 DA06953-03).

[Haworth co-indexing entry note]: "AIDS Risk Behavior in Opioid Dependent Patients Treated with Community Reinforcement Approach and Relationships with Psychiatric Disorders." Abbott, Patrick J. et al. Co-published simultaneously in *Journal of Addictive Diseases* (The Haworth Medical Press, an imprint of The Haworth Press, Inc.) Vol. 17, No. 4, 1998, pp. 33-48; and: *Effects of Substance Abuse Treatment on AIDS Risk Behaviors* (ed: Edward Gottheil, and Barry Stimmel) The Haworth Medical Press, an imprint of The Haworth Press, Inc., 1998, pp. 33-48. Single or multiple copies of this article are available for a fee from The Haworth Document Delivery Service [1-800-342-9678, 9:00 a.m. - 5:00 p.m. (EST). E-mail address: getinfo@haworthpressinc.com].

between comorbid psychiatric disorders and the risk for AIDS behavior in opioid dependent patients entering methadone maintenance treatment. Additionally, we looked at AIDS risk behaviors as they related to the Addition Severity Index (ASI), Beck Depression Inventory, Symptom Checklist-90-Revised (SCL-90-R), and the Social Adjustment Scale-Self Report (SAS-SR). Subjects (N = 227) were drawn from a large clinical trial that examined the effectiveness of a Community Reinforcement Approach for treatment of opioid dependence. Both CRA and standard treatment demonstrated a significant effect on reduction of AIDS risk behaviors. There was no relationship found regarding comorbid psychiatric disorders with the risk for AIDS behavior. However, there were correlations with other psychiatric, social, and substance abuse variables. Multivariate analyses indicated that increased drug and legal ASI composite scores were the primary predictors of increased AIDS risk behavior. *[Article copies available for a fee from The Haworth Document Delivery Service: 1-800-342-9678. E-mail address: getinfo@haworthpressinc.com]*

INTRODUCTION

In 1993, there were 1.3 million injection drug users (IDUs) in the United States with an estimated rate of HIV infection of 25 to 35 percent. This means that there are at least 300,000 to 400,000 HIV-infected IDUs currently in this country.[1] The total number of cases of acquired immunodeficiency syndrome (AIDS) as of December of 1995 reported to the Center for Disease Control was 513,486, of these 184,359 (36%) were directly or indirectly associated with injection-drug use.[2] Worldwide, AIDS cases continue to rise with the major transmission groups being IDUs (37.7%) and homosexual males (35.3%).[3] Not only are IDUs at risk for AIDS, but they expose other populations who would not be at risk otherwise. Even with widespread knowledge of AIDS protection, the problem of HIV transmission among IDUs and associated populations continues unabated. Although IDUs are generally at risk for AIDS due to the infection rates within this population and the route of drug use, it is important to determine additional characteristics of IDUs that are related to higher AIDS risk behaviors so that appropriate interventions to reduce such behavior may be implemented.

There have been several earlier treatment outcome studies that have reported a reduction of drug use behaviors in opioid dependent patients maintained on methadone, but few have looked at change in AIDS risk behaviors.[4,5] We reported in a previous article on 6-month outcome utilizing Community Reinforcement Approach (CRA) in opioid dependent patients on methadone maintenance.[6] In this article we report specifically on CRA's effect on AIDS risk behaviors and relationships to psychiatric disorders and symptoms.

Numerous studies have reported on the prevalence of comorbidity among substance abusers. Data from the Epidemiologic Catchment Area have shown that 64% of patients seeking outpatient treatment for drug abuse have had a psychiatric disorder within the previous six months.[7] Several studies found high rates of pyschopathology in opioid dependent individuals with the most common Axis I diagnosis being major depression and the most frequent Axis II diagnosis being antisocial personality disorder (ASPD).[5,8-12] Additionally, studies have shown that treatment outcome is extensively affected by psychiatric severity and specific comorbid disorders.[4,5,10,13] Further, psychiatric severity has been associated with poor treatment outcome in drug counseling programs.

Recent studies have found relationships between specific psychiatric disorders and increased AIDS risk behavior in opioid addicts. Brooner and his colleagues[12,14] and others[15] have reported increased needle sharing and increased rates of HIV infection in opioid addicts diagnosed with ASPD. Silberstein et al.[11] found a relationship between a primary diagnosis of depression and elevated HIV risk (as indicated by rate of seropositivity) in a group of dually-diagnosed inpatient IDUs. Metzger et al.[16] found that IDUs enrolled in a methadone program who shared needles had significantly higher rates of depression and more severe psychiatric and drug problems than did IDUs who did not share needles. Interestingly, knowledge of preventive measures, fear of contracting AIDS and frequency of injection drug use did not differentiate high and low risk IDUs in Metzger et al.'s study.

The above findings suggest that specific comorbid psychiatric disorders (particularly ASPD and depression) are associated with increased risk for AIDS behaviors. The current study examined whether psychiatric comorbidity in opioid-dependent patients entering treatment was associated with differential risk for AIDS behavior. In addition, we examined whether other variables of psychiatric, social, and substance abuse status were related to AIDS risk behavior.

METHODS

Population

Subjects for this study were taken from a large clinical trial that examined the effectiveness of a Community Reinforcement Approach (CRA) for treatment of heroin addiction. Intravenous drug abusers (N = 227) were recruited between 1991 and 1993 from consecutive admissions to the University of New Mexico's Center on Alcoholism, Substance Abuse and Addictions (CASAA) methadone treatment program. Patients entering the trial had to qualify for methadone maintenance according to Federal Register requirements[17] (21 CFR Part 291) and had to be 18 years of age and have a stable residence in the county. Patients were excluded from the trial if they were acutely psychotic or pregnant, had a significant other in the trial, had been discharged from treatment at the center within the last 6 months, or had gross cognitive impairment.

The sample consisted of 166 (73.1%) males and 61 (26.9%) females. Age ranged from 20 to 63 years with a mean age of 36.71 (SD = 8.55) years and an average of 12.44 (SD = 8.82) years of heroin use. The ethnic/racial composition was 184 (81.1%) Hispanic, 39 (17.2%) White, 3 (1.3%) Native American, and 1 (.04%) Black. Marital status was 55 (24.2%) married, 94 (41.4%) divorced, separated or widowed, and 78 (34.4%) never married. For educational status 74 (32.7%) of the patients had less than a high school education, while 115 (50.7%) had completed high school or the equivalent, 33 (14.5%) had some college, and 3 (1.3%) had a college degree. Within the preceding 3 years 116 (53.7%) had full or part-time employment, 62 (28.7%) had been unemployed, 2 (0.9%) were students, 9 (4.0%) were retired or disabled, and 38 (17.6%) had been incarcerated. Court referrals accounted for almost one fourth of the sample (N = 56). Only 9 individuals (4%) reported that they were homosexual or bisexual.

Measures

The following measures pertinent to psychiatric disorders and risk behavior were obtained for each subject:

Addiction Severity Index (ASI)

The ASI is a structured interview that assesses substance use and related problems.[18] Seven problem areas are covered: Medical Status, Employment Status, Alcohol Use, Drug Use, Legal Status, Family/Social Relationships, and Psychiatric Status. The reliability and validity of the ASI with populations of substance abusers seeking treatment have been demonstrated.[18,19]

Symptom Checklist-90-Revised (SCL-90-R)

The SCL-90-R is a self-administered measure of symptomatic distress, on which respondents rate themselves on a scale ranging from 0-4 for each of the 90 items.[20] Sub-scale scores indicate increasing symptomatic distress in the following areas: (1) somatization; (2) obsessive-compulsivity; (3) interpersonal sensitivity; (4) depression; (5) anxiety; (6) hostility; (7) phobic anxiety; (8) paranoid ideation; and (9) psychoticism. The total score provides an indication of overall psychiatric distress. The reliability and validity of the SCL-90-R as a measure of psychiatric distress has been established. [21,22]

The Beck Depression Inventory (BDI)

The BDI is a 21-item self report questionnaire used to assess the presence and severity of depressive symptoms.[23] Each item is comprised of a group of four statements that describe a range of feelings or experiences. Participants choose the statement that best describes how they have been feeling for the past week. These statements are assigned numerical values (0, 1, 2, and 3) with increasing values representing more depressed feelings or experiences. The reliability and validity of the BDI has been demonstrated.[24]

Risk Assessment Battery (RAB)

The RAB was developed to assess behaviors that place patients at risk for developing HIV and AIDS.[25] This self-administered questionnaire consists of 38 questions which provide 2 sub-scales examining risk for AIDS behavior specific to sexual interaction or injection drug use as well as an overall risk score which ranges from 0 to 1. The reliability and validity of the RAB have been found to be at acceptable levels.[16]

Social Adjustment Scale-Self Report (SAS-SR)

The SAS-SR is a self-administered 54-item questionnaire designed to assess problems with social functioning in nine sub-scales as well as an overall adjustment score.[26] Higher scores are indicative of greater problems with social functioning. The reliability and validity of the SAS-SR has been established.[27]

Structured Clinical Interview for DSM-III-R, Patient Edition (SCID-P)

The SCID-P is a structured, clinical interview for assessing DSM-III-R diagnoses.[28] The SCID-P has demonstrated adequate reliability in diagnosing Axis I disorders.[29] All subjects completed the section for Axis I diagnoses. Subjects were assessed for current and lifetime diagnoses. Current diagnoses were those for which the subjects met criteria within the month prior to assessment. The exceptions to this were dysthymia and generalized anxiety disorder. For those diagnoses, current episode was based on the presence of symptoms over the preceding two-year period for dysthymia and over the preceding six-month period for generalized anxiety disorder. Lifetime diagnoses were those disorders for which the patient met criteria at any point during their lives.

Structured Clinical Interview for DSM-III-R,
Personality Disorders (SCID-II)

The SCID-II is a combined self-administered and interviewer-rated questionnaire that determines the presence of a personality disorder based on DSM-III-R criteria.[30]

Procedures

All subjects were evaluated at the beginning of the clinical treatment trial. The following instruments were completed at intake and at 6, 12, and 18 months: ASI, BDI, SCL-90-R, SAS-SR, and the RAB. The SCID-P and the SCID-II were completed after subjects were in treatment for approximately 1.5 months (Median = 48 days). Assessments were completed by trained master level research assistants. The SCIDs were completed by the following personnel: a psychiatrist, a psychiatric nurse with prior experience and a master level counselor. The master level research assistant completed the majority of the interviews. All interviewers had the following training in the use of the SCID: full day training in the use of the SCID by one of the developers of the instrument (Michael First, M.D.), read the SCID training manual, reviewed the SCID training tapes, and completed several practice interviews. All interviews were audio-taped and 17 of these were diagnosed a second time by a psychiatrist to determine reliability. The level of exact agreement on diagnosis was 59% with a moderate kappa of 0.56.[31]

RESULTS

We examined change in AIDS risk behaviors at 6, 12, and 18 months and whether individuals with specific psychiatric disorders differed from those without such disorders on AIDS risk behaviors. The risk measures were the sub-scale scores of the RAB, the RAB overall score, the presence or absence of reported needle sharing, and whether patients engaged in unprotected sex.

AIDS Risk Behavior

The overall score and both the injection drug use and sexual behavior sub-scales of the RAB showed significant improvement at 6, 12, and 18 months compared to pretreatment levels (all p's < .001, as indicated by repeated measures analysis of variances, ANOVA's). However, there were no significant differences between CRA and Standard interventions in reduction of AIDS risk behaviors.

AIDS Risk and Psychiatric Disorders

There were 227 patients who completed the SCID-P and 200 who completed the SCID-II. Since there were insufficient numbers of many diagnoses to make comparisons, the following diagnoses were chosen for theoretical reasons: lifetime or current diagnoses of any affective disorder, major depression, dysthymia, any anxiety disorder, cocaine and alcohol dependence, ASPD, any Axis I disorder excluding opioid abuse and dependence, and any Axis II disorder. Table 1 presents the number of patients with these disorders.

Risk Assessment Battery

The mean overall risk score for the entire sample was 0.176 (SD = 0.114), while the mean drug risk score was 7.031 (SD = 6.42) and the mean sexual risk score was 4.228 (SD = 2.77). Due to the exploratory nature of the analyses, a larger alpha level of .10 was chosen. However, since there were repeated test on the same dependent measures (sexual risk, drug risk, and overall risk), Bonferroni adjusted comparisons were used by dividing the

TABLE 1. Lifetime and Current Rates of Psychiatric Diagnoses in Opioid Addicts

Diagnosis	Lifetime		Current	
	N	%	N	%
Any Affect Disorder	70	31.0	39	17.0
Major Depression	51	22.5	14	6.0
Dysthymia	28	12.0	28	12.0
Any Anxiety Disorder	33	14.5	22	10.0
Cocaine Dependence	99	49.5	28	12.0
Alcohol Dependence	126	56.0	15	7.0
ASPD	62	31.0	62	31.0
Any Axis I Disorder	181	80.0	109	48.0
Any Axis II Disorder	84	42.0	84	42.0

alpha level among the number of comparisons examined (.10/15). Thus, any specific test needed to be significant at the .0067 alpha level. We first compared subjects with any of the psychiatric diagnoses listed in Table 1 with individuals without that disorder (including any Axis I disorder or any Axis II disorder) on the RAB. We examined three dependent variables of the RAB: sexual risk, drug risk, and overall risk. There were no differences in any of the measures of AIDS risk between patients with a specific disorder compared to those without that disorder. This conclusion was not based solely on the use of the restricted alpha level since only one test (of 30) indicated a significance level less than the traditional .05 (specifically, .043) which would be expected by chance alone.

Needle Sharing and Unprotected Sex

In addition to examining the 3 continuous scores of the RAB, we also examined whether patients reported sharing needles with others (Question #14 of the RAB). There were 133 individuals that reported that they had shared a needle or works at least once in the last 6 months, and 95 individuals reported that they had not shared or had not used in the past 6 months. As with the continuous measures, we examined all of the DSM-III-R diagnoses listed in Table 1, including any lifetime or current Axis I disorder (excluding opioid abuse and dependence) and any lifetime or current Axis II disorder. Again we used protected tests to examine whether needle sharers were more likely to have these diagnoses. As with the continuous measures, no SCID diagnosis was more or less prevalent for needle sharers than non-needle sharers, nor did the general categories of any Axis 1 or Axis II diagnoses show reliable differences. In fact, the results regarding any current Axis I diagnosis was in the opposite direction of expectation in that only 44% of needle sharers had a current Axis I diagnosis compared to 54% of non-needle sharers.

Whether patients reported having unprotected sex in the last 6 months was also examined, based on question 34 of the RAB. One hundred and fifty-nine individuals reported having unprotected sex at least once in the past six months, while 68 reported none or only protected sex. As with the findings regarding needle sharing, none of the diagnostic categories listed in Table 1 were found to be significantly associated with unprotected sex.

AIDS Risk and Other Variables

We also examined whether other variables were related either individually or in combination with the RAB. We conducted correlations (presented in Table 2) and multiple regressions of the ASI composite scores, the BDI, and

TABLE 2. Correlations of RAB Scores with Substance Use, Social Interaction, and Psychiatric Functioning Variables

	Mean (SD)	Drug Risk	Sex Risk	Total Risk
ASI Variables				
Medical	0.24 (0.34)	− 0.07	0.005	− 0.06
Employment	0.68 (0.28)	0.15	− 0.06	0.11
Alcohol	0.10 (0.18)	0.13	0.06	0.13
Drug	0.30 (0.11)	0.26*	0.15	0.28*
Legal	0.17 (0.23)	0.26*	0.14	0.28*
Family/Social	0.18 (0.23)	0.00	0.14	0.05
Psychological	0.19 (0.21)	− 0.04	0.02	0.05
SAS-SR Variables				
Work Outside Home	1.98 (1.27)	0.12	0.12	0.15
Social & Leisure	2.57 (0.73)	0.14	0.08	0.15
Extended Family	1.90 (0.74)	0.22*	0.13	0.25*
Marital	0.98 (1.00)	0.15	0.13	0.18
Parental	0.74 (0.89)	− 0.05	0.17	0.02
Family Unit	1.95 (1.15)	0.14	0.08	0.16
Economic	3.23 (1.54)	0.21*	0.07	0.22*
Overall Adjustment	2.17 (0.59)	0.22*	0.12	0.24*
SCL-90-R Variables				
Somatization	9.87 (8.72)	0.12	0.02	0.11
Obsessive-Compulsive	8.15 (7.49)	0.13	− 0.04	0.10
Int-Sensitivity	5.62 (6.00)	0.15	0.01	0.14
Depression	12.02 (10.65)	0.19*	0.06	0.19*
Anxiety	6.77 (6.93)	0.15	− 0.01	0.13
Hostility	3.74 (4.56)	0.15	− 0.005	0.13
Phobic Anxiety	2.70(4.15)	0.14	−0.04	0.11
Paranoid Ideation	3.93 (4.15)	0.15	0.02	0.14
Psychoticism	4.32 (5.78)	0.16	0.07	0.12
Additional	6.76 (5.57)	0.17	− 0.07	0.18
Positive Symptom Total	36.93 (24.76)	0.23*	0.01	0.20*
BDI	13.93 (10.31)	0.17	0.09	0.19*
*significant at adjusted alpha level (p < .009)				

the SCL-90-R and the SAS-SR with the three variables of the RAB. Likewise, we did similar analyses of needle sharing and unprotected sex with the same variables.

Risk Assessment Battery

Again protected tests were used, resulting in an alpha level for each correlation of .009 (.10/11). Table 2 presents the mean intake values of the continuous variables examined and the simple correlations between these measures and the RAB scores. As can be seen in the Table, there were few significant correlations, and of those only a few were of moderate strength. The sexual risk variable was not significantly correlated with any of the variables tested. On the ASI the only variables that indicated a significant relationship with the RAB were the drug and legal composite scores. The drug composite score correlated significantly with drug risk and overall risk. The legal composite score also correlated with drug risk and overall risk. Both of these variables indicated that as drug and legal problems increased, risk behavior for AIDS increased.

As noted above, the SAS-SR has 9 sub-scales and an overall score. The Student and Work at Home sub-scales were based on very few subjects (N = 3, and 19 respectively) and therefore were not examined. For the drug risk scale the overall SAS-SR score correlated significantly such that increased social adjustment problems were associated with increased drug risk. Subsequent analysis of the sub-scale correlations indicated that increased economic and extended family problems predicted increased drug risk. The same pattern was shown for the overall risk score. Increased social adjustment problems were directly related to general risk, and the significant follow-ups were for the extended family and economic sub-scales were related in the bivariate relationships.

For the SCL-90-R the Positive Symptom Total correlated with drug risk and overall risk such that increases in positive symptoms were directly associated with increases in reported risk behavior. Follow-up analyses of the sub-scales indicated that the only significant relationship was with the depression sub-scale which correlated with drug risk as well as overall risk. This significant correlation was replicated with the BDI indicating that increased depressive symptoms were associated with increased AIDS risk behavior.

We conducted multiple regression analyses to determine what combination of variables would predict overall risk behavior. Two different analyses were conducted. The first approach used all subjects in a standard stepwise regression, while the second analysis used a double cross-validation technique. Since multiple regression can capitalize on chance variables being included in an overall regression equation, the double cross-validation approach is a means of protecting against sample specific fluctuations so that the resulting equation can be a better indicator of population predictors.[32]

For the overall stepwise regression we entered all of the composite scores for the ASI, the sub-scales from the SCL-90-R and the SAS-SR, and the BDI. The overall scores from the SCL-90-R and the SAS-SR were not included since they would be highly correlated with the sub-scales and would be less theoretically meaningful (although the results were similar when the overall scores were used instead of the sub-scales). There were five significant predictors of overall RAB scores ($p < .05$). These were the drug and legal composite scores from the ASI and the economic, marital, and social sub-scales of the SAS-SR. Each variable entered in this order. The equation was:

$$RAB = .2093*DRUG + .1056*LEGAL + .0096*ECON + .0160*MARITAL + .0200*SOCIAL.$$

The multiple correlation coefficient was 0.45, $F(5,213) = 10.68$, $p < .0001$, indicating that 20% of the variability in RAB scores was accounted for by these variables.

For the double cross-validation procedure patients were randomly divided into two groups. We then conducted stepwise multiple regression using all continuous variables on one of the two samples. This resulted in a single equation that included the significant variables for predicting RAB scores for that sample. We then used these same variables to predict RAB scores for the second half of the population. Variables that significantly predicted in both samples were considered reliable predictors and the equation for these variables were determined for the entire population. The cross validation approach entered all of the variables mentioned above into the stepwise regression. The variables that were significant for the first sample (and entered the equation in this order) were the marital sub-scale from the SAS-SR, the legal composite from the ASI, the family unit sub-scale from the SAS-SR, and the family-social sub-scale from the SAS-SR, $F(4,103) = 6.57$, $p = .0001$ ($r = .451$). The only variable that was a significant predictor when these variables were entered for the second sample was the legal composite score.

If a more lenient criteria for significance is used across the two samples ($p < .10$), then a second variable of the ASI drug composite score combined with the legal composite score was a significant predictor across the two samples. The equation for these two predictors for the entire sample was:

$$RAB = .240* DRUG + .110* LEGAL$$

This equation significantly predicted RAB scores, $F(2,216) = 16.59$, $p < .0001$, with a multiple correlation of 0.365, thus accounting for approximately 13.3% of the variability in RAB score. These findings suggest that within this population of New Mexico heroin users, both drug and legal problems are the primary predictors for AIDS risk behavior. This is consistent with the univariate results in that these variables both had moderate simple correlations with RAB scores.

Needle Sharers vs. Non-Needle Sharers

Again we used protected tests to examine whether needle sharers differed from non-needle sharers on the continuous variables of the ASI, SCL-90-R, SAS-SR, and BDI. No variables of the SCL-90-R, the SAS-SR, or the BDI indicated any significantly different means for sharers compared to non-sharers. However, on the ASI the tests of the drug and legal composites were significant. This indicated that needle sharers had more drug (M = .32, SD = .09) and legal problems (M = .23, SD = .24) than non-needle sharers (M = .27, SD = .12 for drug and M = .11, SD = .19 for legal).

Discriminant function analyses were conducted to determine whether a linear combination of variables would distinguish between needle sharers and non-needle sharers. As was done with the multiple regression, we conducted a discriminant function analysis for the entire population and a double cross-validation using one half of the subjects as one sample and the other half for the other sample. The overall discriminant function analysis examined all of the ASI composite scores, the SCL-90-R sub-scales, the SAS-SR sub-scales, and the BDI. Of all these variables, five differentiated needle sharers from non-needle sharers. These were the legal composite score, the drug composite score, the *inverse* of the family/social composite score, and the interpersonal sensitivity sub-scale of the SCL-90-R. Each of these variables significantly contributed to the discriminant function, and the overall function significantly differentiated needle sharers from non-needle sharers, $F(4,214) = 7.56$, $p<.0001$. The standardized canonical discriminant functions were 0.695 for the legal composite score, 0.525 for the drug composite score, -0.507 for the family/social composite score, and 0.407 for the interpersonal sensitivity sub-scale. The canonical correlation for the function was 0.35, suggesting that approximately 12% of the variability between needle sharers and non-needle sharers was due to this linear combination of variables. The double cross-validation approach indicated no variables that reliably distinguished between sharers and non-sharers for both samples.

Unprotected Sex

Consistent with the findings for the sexual risk sub-scale, there were no significant differences between patients who reported having unprotected sex compared to those who reported none or only protected sex on the continuous measures of the ASI composite scores, SCL-90-R, SAS-SR, and BDI. Discriminant function analyses also indicated no differences due to unprotected sex.

DISCUSSION

We demonstrated a clear benefit for both the CRA and standard interventions in reduction of AIDS risk behavior for opioid dependent patients on methadone maintenance. For both the CRA and standard interventions, overall risk and both injection and sexual risk behaviors improved; injection risk behaviors improved to a greater degree. Although there were no differences between treatment conditions in outcome on the RAB, CRA was more effective than standard treatment on other outcome variables in an earlier study.[6]

There was no relationship in this study of psychiatric disorders (as determined by the SCID-P and SCID-II) with risk for AIDS behavior. However, there were correlations with other psychiatric, social, and substance abuse variables. Univariate analyses demonstrated that the drug and legal composite scores of the ASI as well as the overall score of the SAS-SR, BDI, and SCL-90-R correlated with the overall score of the RAB. Similarly, multivariate analyses showed that the primary relationships were between the ASI legal and drug composite scores with the RAB drug risk sub-scale and overall scores. In other words, both drug and legal problems for this sample of opioid-dependent individuals were primary predictors of AIDS risk behaviors; individuals with more drug and legal problems were at higher risk for AIDS risk behaviors.

Further, we examined needle sharing and unprotected sexual behavior in this population and our findings were similar although less strong. Although unprotected sex was unrelated to the variables examined, patients who reported sharing needles in the past 6 months showed higher levels of drug and legal problems (higher legal and drug composite scores). The discriminant function analyses suggested that needle sharers as compared to non-needle sharers had more legal and drug problems, more interpersonal sensitivity, and fewer family/social problems, although this was not confirmed using the cross-validation approach.

Our results differ from our preliminary findings as well as the results of other investigators in that we found no relationship between AIDS risk behaviors and specific psychiatric disorders.[8,14,15] Other groups have found a relationship with ASPD. In addition, our preliminary report suggested that dysthymic individuals showed higher levels of risk. The exception to this is a recent study by McCusker et al.[33] who, similar to our study, found no relationship of AIDS risk behaviors with psychiatric disorders. This may be attributed to differences in the characteristics and settings of the populations examined which may alter patterns of risk taking behaviors. Our population was largely Hispanic (81.1%) and none of the patients in the study were HIV positive. This is consistent with low rates of HIV positive patients in individuals that present to treatment in New Mexico.[34] In addition, only 4% of our population reported that they were homosexual or bisexual. There were also differences in the instruments and criteria used to arrive at a psychiatric diagnosis; Brooner and his colleagues used Research Diagnostic Criteria that are more restrictive in focus than DSM-III-R criteria particularly for ASPD.

However, our findings partially replicated Metzger et al.'s[16] results. They found increased AIDS risk behaviors in individuals with higher scores on the SCL-90-R and BDI and with the ASI drug and legal composite scores. We did not find the correlation with the ASI psychiatric composite scores that Metzger et al. found.

There were limitations in our study. The study was designed as a treatment trial and not specifically designed to investigate the relationship between psychiatric disorders and AIDS risk behaviors. It was only at the completion of the treatment trial that we chose to look at this relationship. However, most of the prior work in this area had similar designs and were embedded in clinical treatment trials. Additionally, the SCID-II may not be the ideal instrument to diagnose ASPD, using criteria that may be overly inclusive. Finally, as stated above, our population was largely Hispanic and unique to New Mexico, therefore, these findings may not generalize to other populations. Further, the rate of cumulative AIDS cases in New Mexico related to exposure to injection drug use is less than 7%, and one survey of injection drug users in Albuquerque found only .08% of individuals positive for HIV.[34] This is at great variance with other regions of the country and other infectious diseases in New Mexico that have similar routes of transmission as HIV, such as Hepatitis B and C that were positive in 66.7% and 89%, respectively, of individuals in the same population.[34] Why there is such a discrepancy is not entirely clear. In part this has been explained by lack of mobility of this population and that injection drug use occurs in relatively closed social networks.

Clearly, it is important to identify subgroups of patients in methadone treatment programs that are at higher risk for AIDS behavior so that these individuals can be targeted for specific preventive interventions. The risk factors and related treatment interventions will vary depending on the region of the country. In New Mexico patients with more severe legal and drug problems as measured by the ASI are engaging in behavior that places them at higher risk of developing serious infectious diseases, specifically AIDS and hepatitis. Methadone treatment programs need to develop additional services to both identify and reduce risk behavior, and these services must be tailored for the unique populations they serve.

REFERENCES

1. Des Jarlais DC. Cross-national studies of AIDS among injecting drug users. Addiction. 1994; 89:383-392.

2. Centers for Disease Control: HIV/AIDS Surveillance Report, Vol.6,2. Washington, DC, Department of Health and Human Services: Fall 1995.

3. Wodak AD, Crofts N, Fisher R. HIV infection among injecting drug users in Asia: An evolving public health crisis. AIDS Care. 1993; 22:549-562.

4. McLellan AT, Luborsky L, Woody GE, et al. Predicting response to alcohol and drug abuse treatments: role of psychiatric severity. Arch Gen Psychiatry. 1983; 40:620-625.

5. Woody GE, Luborsky L, McLellan AT, et al. Psychotherapy for opiate addicts: Does it help? Arch Gen Psychiatry. 1983; 40:639-645.

6. Abbot PA, Weller SB, Delaney HD, Moore BA. Community Reinforcement Approach in the treatment of opiate addiction. Am J Drug Alcohol Abuse. (In Press)

7. Reiger D, Farmer M, Rae D. Comorbidity of mental disorders with alcohol and other drug abuse: Results from the Epidemiologic Catchment Area study. JAMA. 1990; 264:2511-2518.

8. Abbott PA, Weller SB, Walker SR. Psychiatric disorders of opioid addicts entering treatment: Preliminary data. J Addict. 1994; 13:1-11.

9. Khantzian EJ, Treece C. DSM-III psychiatric diagnosis of narcotic addicts: Recent findings. Arch Gen Psychiatry. 1985; 42:1067-1071.

10. Rounsaville BJ, Weissman MM, Kleber H, Wilber C. Heterogeneity of psychiatric diagnosis in treated opiate addicts. Arch Gen Psychiatry. 1982; 39:161-166.

11. Silberstein C, Galanter M, Marmor M, et al. HIV-1 among inner city dually diagnosed inpatients. Am J Drug Alcohol Abuse. 1994; 20:101-113.

12. Brooner RK, Greenfield L, Schmidt CW, Bigelow GE. Antisocial personality disorder and HIV infection among intravenous drug abusers. Am J Psychiatry. 1993; 150:53-58.

13. Rounsaville BJ, Kosten TR, Weissman MM, Kleber HD. Prognostic significance of psychopathology in treated opiate addicts: A 2.5-year follow-up study. Arch Gen Psychiatry. 1986; 43:739-745.

14. Brooner RK, Bigelow GE, Strain E, Schmidt CW. Intravenous drug abusers with antisocial personality disorder: Increased HIV risk behavior. Drug Alcohol Depend. 1990; 26:39-44.

15. Gill K, Nolimal D, Crowley TJ. Antisocial personality disorder, HIV risk behavior and retention in methadone maintenance therapy. Drug Alcohol Depend. 1992; 30:247-252.

16. Metzger DS, Woody GE, De Philippis D, et al. Risk factors for needle sharing among methadone-treated patients. Am J Psychiatry. 1991; 148:636-640.

17. Federal Register, Part III, 54, (40), 21 CFR Part 291, Rockville, MD: US Department of Health and Human Services, Food and Drug Administration: 1989.

18. McLellan AT, Luborsky L, Cacciola J, et al. New data from the Addiction Severity Index: Reliability and validity in three centers. J Nerv Ment Dis. 1985; 173:412-423.

19. Kosten TR, Rounsaville BJ, Kleber HD. Concurrent validity of the Addition Severity Index. J Nerv Ment Dis. 1983; 171:606-610.

20. Derogatis LR. SCL-90-R: Administration, scoring and procedures manual II. Rockville, MD: Clinical Psychometric Research, 1983.

21. Derogatis LR, Cleary PA. Confirmation of the dimensional structure of the SCL-90. A study in construct validation. J Clin Psychol. 1977; 33:981-989.

22. Derogatis LR, Cleary PA. Factorial invariance across gender for the primary symptom dimensions of the SCL-90. Brit J Soc Clin Psychol. 1977; 16:347-356.

23. Beck AT, Ward CH, Mendelson M, et al. An inventory for measuring depression. Arch Gen Psychiatry. 1961; 4:53-63.

24. Beck AT. Depression inventory. Philadelphia, PA: Center for Cognitive Therapy. 1978.

25. Metzger DS, De Phillips D, Druley P, et al. The impact of HIV testing on risk of AIDS behaviors. Problems of drug dependence 1991: Proceeding of the 53rd Annual Scientific Meeting. NIDA Res Monogr, 119. 1992; 297-298.

26. Weissman MM, Bothwell S. Assessment of social adjustment by patient self-report. Arch Gen Psychiatry. 1976; 33:1111-1115.

27. Weissman MM, Paykel ES, Prusoff BA. Social adjustment scale handbook: Rationale, reliability, and validity. 1990.

28. Spitzer RL, Williams JBW, Gibbon M, First B. Structured clinical interview for DSM-III-R patient version (SCID-P, 6/1/88). New York: Biometrics Research Department, State Psychiatric Institute, 1988.

29. Williams JBW, Gibbon M, First B, Spitzer RL. The Structured Clinical Interview for DSM-III-R (SCID): II. Multisite test-retest reliability. Arch Gen Psychiatry. 1992; 49:630-636.

30. Spitzer RL, Williams JBW, Gibbon M, First B. User's guide for the structured clinical interview for DSM-III-R (SCID). Washington, DC: American Psychiatric Press, 1990.

31. Cohen J. A coefficient of agreement of nominal scales. Educ Psychol Meas. 1960; 20:37-46.

32. Mosier CI. Problems and designs of cross-validation. Educ Psychol Meas. 1960; 11:5-11.

33. McCusker J, Golstein R, Bigelow C, Zorn M. Psychiatric status and HIV risk reduction among residential drug abuse treatment clients. Addiction. 1995; 90:1377-1387.

34. New Mexico Department of Health, Division of Epidemiology, Evaluation and Planning. Epidemiology report, High prevalence of hepatitis and low prevalence of HIV among injection drug users in Bernalillo and Dona Ana counties. July 1995.

Assessment of HIV Risk

Marek C. Chawarski, PhD
Juliana Pakes
Richard S. Schottenfeld, MD

SUMMARY. Based on the review of existing instruments and analysis of problems encounted in clinical and research practice with one of the most commonly used assessment instruments, the RAB, this paper proposes a number of solutions aimed at improving validity, and efficiency of assessment of HIV risk in drug abusing populations. Briefly, five domains of assessment are discussed: intravenous drug use, high-risk sexual behaviors, knowledge of HIV transmission and methods of prevention, psychological aspects of behavioral change, and epidemiological factors of HIV transmission. The paper discusses also changes in format, scope, and context, as well as scoring procedures that may improve discriminability and sensitivity to detect change of a comprehensive HIV risk assessment instrument. Finally, a process of developing an HIV risk assessment instrument, the ARI-I, which is based on the proposed recommendations and which incorporates methodological improvements discussed in the paper is briefly described. *[Article copies available for a fee from The Haworth Document Delivery Service: 1-800-342-9678. E-mail address: getinfo@haworthpressinc.com]*

INTRODUCTION

Drug abuse has emerged as the leading factor associated with transmission of the human immunodeficiency virus (HIV) in many urban settings in the

Marek C. Chawarski, Juliana Pakes, and Richard S. Schottenfeld are all affiliated with the Substance Abuse Center, Department of Psychiatry, Yale University School of Medicine.

Address correspondence to: Marek C. Chawarski, PhD, Yale University, Department of Psychiatry, CMHC/SAC, Suite S214, 34 Park Street, New Haven, CT 06519.

[Haworth co-indexing entry note]: "Assessment of HIV Risk." Chawarski, Marek C., Juliana Pakes, and Richard S. Schottenfeld. Co-published simultaneously in *Journal of Addictive Diseases* (The Haworth Medical Press, an imprint of The Haworth Press, Inc.) Vol. 17, No. 4, 1998, pp. 49-59; and: *Effects of Substance Abuse Treatment on AIDS Risk Behaviors* (ed: Edward Gottheil, and Barry Stimmel) The Haworth Medical Press, an imprint of The Haworth Press, Inc., 1998, pp. 49-59. Single or multiple copies of this article are available for a fee from The Haworth Document Delivery Service [1-800-342-9678, 9:00 a.m. - 5:00 p.m. (EST). E-mail address: getinfo@haworthpressinc.com].

U.S., particularly among women.[1,2] HIV infections followed by the Acquired Immunodeficiency Syndrome (AIDS) are also the leading cause of mortality among drug dependent persons.[3] Both epidemiological data and clinical studies[4-7] show an association between alcohol and drug abuses and HIV infections. Although factors affecting the onset and spread of HIV infection and the development of AIDS in this population are only partially understood, behaviors associated with intravenous injections of drugs (for drug injectors), and complex behavioral connections between drug use and sexual practices (for both injectors and non-injectors) are critical.[2,8-17]

Because of the association between drug abuse and HIV transmission, modification of high-risk behavioral patterns among drug-abusing populations is a major focus of drug abuse treatment and research.[18-20] Although reduction of the risk of HIV transmission is a key outcome measure regarding the effectiveness of drug-abuse treatment, methods for reliable and valid assessment of behaviors associated with high risk of HIV infection and changes in risk behaviors are not well developed.[21,22]

Only a limited number of HIV risk-assessment instruments are available, and to our knowledge, no single comprehensive review of instruments for assessing risk of HIV infection has been published. The NIDA AIDS Initial Assessment Questionnaire (AIA) (NOVA Research Company, 1989), the HIV Risk Taking Behaviour Scale (HRBS),[23] and the Risk for AIDS Behavior (RAB)[24] are among the most commonly used in the field of drug abuse. Problems with these and other instruments include their lack of sufficiently established psychometric properties and their limited coverage of all relevant domains of risk.[25,26]

In this paper, we describe our analysis of the limitations of one widely used HIV risk assessment instrument, the RAB. Based on problems that we identified in using this instrument in our clinical and research practice, we set out to develop an improved risk assessment instrument by (1) reviewing literature to identify key domains of risk, (2) constructing and pilot testing a prototype HIV risk assessment instrument, and (3) based on the results of our pilot testing, revising the risk domains and identifying central methodological problems in assessing risk of HIV infection in drug abusing population. In this paper, we present an overview of our process of identifying important problems associated with the measurement of HIV risk behaviors, and the solutions to these problems that emerged during developing and testing a prototype of an improved assessment instrument.

EVALUATION OF THE RAB

The Risk for AIDS Behavior (RAB) has been used in clinical trials conducted at the Substance Abuse Center at Yale University as one measure for assessing risk of HIV infection. To evaluate the sensitivity of this instrument to detect change in behavioral patterns associated with risk of HIV infection, we analyzed the response characteristics of the RAB among 273 subjects enrolled in clinical trials at the SAC between January 1994 and May 1996. The strong clustering of the results at the low end of the scale and limited variability of scores suggests that the RAB may not be sufficiently sensitive to detect a change in the pattern of behaviors indicating a change in the level of subjects' risk of HIV infection during treatment.

A plot of the frequency distribution of the RAB scores from 273 subjects and basic descriptive measures of central tendency show that the majority of the RAB scores fell into the low end of the scale. The mean (SD) of the RAB scores for the population of 273 subjects was RAB score = 6.3 (5.37), where a possible range of scores is between 0 and 64 (see also Figure 1).

Our analysis also showed limited variability and low rates of positive responses to selected items of the RAB (e.g., sharing needles without cleaning, sharing needles with someone who has AIDS, going to a "shooting gallery," or engaging in unprotected sex with someone who has AIDS). Although such a pattern of responses may reflect current attitudes and behavioral patterns among the population of drug abusers due to extensive HIV education and outreach, it also indicates a limited sensitivity of the assess-

FIGURE 1. Frequency Distribution of the RAB Scores in the Population of 273 Drug Abusing Subjects in Drug Treatment Program.

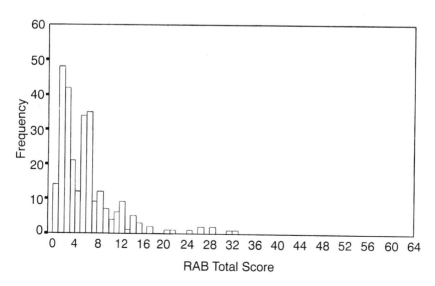

ment instrument to detect differences among subjects or changes in behavior over time.

We also compared the RAB scores for subjects with known HIV positive serologic status and subjects who tested negative for HIV. The difference between the mean of the RAB score for these two groups of subjects was small and statistically not significant (F $(1,267)$ = 0.6, non-significant), indicating that any current or lifetime differences in risk behaviors between these two groups are not detected by the RAB (see also Table 1).

Further review of the RAB identified additional problems with the RAB scoring procedures. The RAB, as well as many other assessment instruments, use aggregate measures of behaviors (e.g., "In the past three months, how often have you used needles after someone else?"). Although such aggregate measures can provide some indication of the client's level of risk of HIV infection, they can also be misleading. One problem is that it may be difficult for the clients to provide information in an aggregate fashion–e.g., as an overall frequency of sharing a cotton in the past three months–especially if such information regards behaviors occurring irregularly or behaviors related to situations in which clients are under the influence of drugs or alcohol. An alternative indication of the frequency of a given behavior is information about the most recent occurrence of such behavior, which is usually easier to recall by the client. The combination of the recency and the frequency of behaviors within a given period, say, one month, may be the most accurate indication of the level of risk associated with these behaviors.

A second problem with aggregate measures is that risk associated with many behaviors may be context dependent. For example, a person who shares injecting equipment or refrains from condom use with a spouse but does not engage in these behaviors with anyone else may be at lower risk of HIV infection, assuming that both partners have the same seropositive status, than a person who sporadically shares injecting equipment or has unprotected sex with strangers, unknown, or casual partners. Our own research data also indicate different patterns of sexual behaviors with steady partners and with

TABLE 1. Comparison of the RAB scores for subjects with different HIV status.

HIV Status	Mean RAB Score (SD)	N
Negative	6.23 (4.89)	230
Positive	6.95 (7.78)	39
Never got the results	6.25 (4.35)	4

strangers or "trade" partners. A risk assessment instrument should include mechanisms for differentiating between different contexts in which behaviors occur. For example, different sets of questions should be included regarding on the one hand sexual practices with a spouse, mate, or a steady partner, and on the other hand sexual practices with strangers or "trade" partners.

Finally, some behaviors associated with sharing of injecting equipment and high-risk sex behaviors have been widely publicized in the media as responsible for HIV infection so that currently the number of clients reporting them is very small. For example, in our recent studies, no clients reported sharing injecting equipment or having unprotected sex with a person infected with the HIV virus, which is an item on the RAB. It is not clear, however, whether this low rate reflects actual behavior or client's reluctance to report highly stigmatized behavior. Validity of self-reported data is a critical issue for all assessment instruments, and, as discussed below, assessments can be designed to help evaluate validity.

DOMAINS FOR ASSESSMENT

Based on the problems with the RAB, we reviewed existing assessment instruments and literature related to HIV risk to identify key domains for inclusion in assessment instrument and to identify strategies for effective and reliable collection of information related to these domains of assessment. Many of the initial assessments instruments focused predominantly on the domains of injection equipment sharing and sexual practices with gay or bisexual men. Although these were the first groups of behaviors identified as responsible for HIV transmission, more recent studies have identified a larger number of other important factors. Among them are unsafe heterosexual practices, such as trading sex for drugs or money; sex with strangers, unknown or casual partners; and group sex, especially under drug or alcohol influence; as well as using and sharing of injecting equipment in larger groups of people ("Shooting Gallery") and sharing of injecting equipment and trading sex when traveling to different parts of the country or abroad (see also[27,28]). Higher rates of HIV infection among crack or freebase cocaine users[29,30] are unrelated to injection drug use; the most probable causes of these increased rates are related to drug effects on psycho-social functioning, including sexual stimulation, increased sex drive, and disinhibition, and cultural features associated with drug use (e.g., drugs and sex parties and trading sex for drugs). Although there have been no studies comparing the relative risk of all these various risk behaviors, a comprehensive instrument for assessment of risk of HIV infection need to include all these relevant domains.

Our review of existing assessment instruments and the relevant literature suggests five major domains associated with high risk of HIV infection that should be included in a comprehensive assessment instrument. These domains are: (1) factors associated with use of contaminated drug injection equipment, (2) factors associated with high-risk sexual behaviors, (3) knowledge of epidemiological and biological factors associated with HIV transmission, and methods of prevention of HIV infection, (4) motivation to reduce risk and other psychological factors affecting the likelihood of maintaining behavioral changes, such as locus of control, impulsivity, risk-taking, and thrill seeking behaviors, and (5) history of other infectious diseases, such as tuberculosis (TB), hepatitis, and sexually transmitted diseases (STD) (see [31,32]). Only the first two domains are commonly represented in risk assessment instruments. However, both knowledge about HIV transmission and its prevention, and a motivation to change behavioral patterns are necessary to modify behavior and to reduce the risk of HIV infection, and information about the history of other infectious diseases can provide additional, indirect indication of the actual level of risk even in the absence of direct indicators, such as needle sharing or unprotected sex with high-risk partners.

While many assessment instruments utilize a standard questionnaire format requiring responses on all items in the instrument, a tree-like structure, as used in the Structured Clinical Interview for DSM-IV (SCID)[33] allows more efficient and in-depth assessment of the risk based on domains of risk representative of each individual. Instruments using a tree-like structure ask broad screening questions related to each important domain and allow in-depth assessment of the domains with positive responses to the screening questions. Such an approach allows detection of behavioral patterns that are characteristic for individual clients and more extensive investigation of them, whereas behaviors that are not present for a person are omitted from further questioning or investigated to a lesser extent. Such a tree-like structure of questioning eliminates the unnecessary burden of asking multiple questions related to factors that are either not present in the behavioral patterns of a given client, or that client denies. This approach also allows assessment of the level of risk for each client on the basis of the combination of factors that are common or typical for some individual clients but are not necessarily common or typical for a larger population.

For example, women who smoke cocaine or crack may not use or share drug injecting equipment and may not report sexual contacts with gay or bisexual men. Asking a series of questions about sharing of the injecting equipment poses unnecessary burden on this group of clients. High-risk sexual behaviors, however, should be investigated more extensively in this group of clients, since they may be trading sex for drugs or money or having unprotected sex with multiple high risk partners. Summarizing briefly, a comprehensive risk assessment instrument should be able to detect as many as possible factors related to high-risk of HIV infection without being unnecessarily time consuming and burdensome for the clients, and the tree-like structure with a broad spectrum of screening questions and a built-in mechanism for in-depth questioning of domains typical for each client represent an excellent solution.

Finally, the stigma associated with many high risk behaviors may lead patients to deny their actual behaviors. The problem may be addressed by assessing high risk behaviors not only by direct questions but also by indirect questions or measures. For example, questions regarding number of needles and syringes used, and the number of contraceptives (condoms) used in a given time period, and the information about the number of sex partners in combination with information about frequency of the related behaviors may provide more accurate information about the actual level of use of precautions. Similarly, the client's history of other infectious diseases, especially sexually transmitted diseases, tuberculosis, and hepatitis can be an indirect indication of the actual level of HIV risk. Finally, a brief visual inspection to detect track marks may be useful to validate reports regarding injection use.[34]

DEVELOPMENT OF THE ARI-I

Based on the considerations discussed above, we developed a structured interview, called the AIDS Risk Inventory (ARI-I), to assess the risk of HIV infection in a population of drug abusers. Our goal was to develop a method that not will only allow quantification of behaviors associated with risk of HIV infection, but will also be sensitive to detect change in the level of risk of HIV infection during treatment.

The original version of the ARI-I was a structured interview containing questions about behaviors associated with drug use, sexual practices, and general knowledge of AIDS prevention. To allow quantification of risk behaviors and detection of their changes, the ARI-I investigates both frequency and recency of the behaviors associated with high risk of HIV infection. Additionally, a "tree-like" structure of the ARI-I allows in-depth testing of high-risk behaviors that are client-specific. All life-time occurrences of high-risk behaviors reported by a client during the interview are further explored by asking questions about the most recent occurrence and the frequency of this behavior during the past three months, omitting questions regarding behaviors not reported by the client.

Several preliminary versions of the ARI have been pilot tested on approximately 300 subjects from two groups of substance abusers: (a) cocaine dependent women, and (b) agonist maintained men and women, to evaluate the feasibility of its administration in clinical research settings, its acceptability to patients, its ability to discriminate between subjects with high and low risk of HIV infection, and its response characteristics. The most recent version of the instrument contains 50 questions divided into three sections.

The Drug Use Section contains 12 questions that investigate a group of behaviors associated with intravenous injection of drugs, such as needle sharing and needle cleaning.

The Sexual Practices Section contains 27 questions divided into two parts investigating: (a) sex practices with a steady/current sex partner, and (b) sex practices with any other, either current or past, sex partner. Since the pattern of sex practices with a steady partner may be different from similar behaviors with casual sex partners, the Sexual Practices Section investigates the following groups of behaviors: (a) engaging in sex while on drugs or alcohol, (b) trading sex for drugs, money, or gifts, (c) engaging in sex with intravenous drug users, (d) engaging in casual sex with unknown people, and (e) use of condoms for all of the above sexual activities.

Calculation of the ARI-I score is based on the frequency of occurrence of a given behavior and on the recency of this behavior, with recency being weighted more than a life-time occurrence of the same behavior. Therefore, the frequency of behaviors associated with drug use and sexual practices during the past three months contributes most to the total score of ARI-I. The present method of scoring is designed to increase the sensitivity of the ARI-I to detect a recent change, or change during treatment, in subjects' behavioral patterns of drug use and sex practices that are associated with high-risk of HIV infection. In the future, we plan to employ discriminant analysis to secure optimum weights for distinguishing among targeted groups of subjects. Standardization of the ARI-I has not yet been established.

The last section of the ARI-I is currently under revision, with plans to expand it to three sections. In the next revision of the ARI-I, we plan to include: (a) a section regarding a history of sexually transmitted and other infectious diseases, (b) a section regarding knowledge of HIV transmission and prevention, and (c) a section pertaining to motivation to change risk behaviors and other psychological factors affecting behavior change. We are currently working on selection of items for these sections. Due to its experimental state, newer versions of the ARI-I may contain changes in both the number and the content of the questions in each of the five sections.

CONCLUSIONS

In summary, the results of pilot testing show that the ARI-I can be successfully used in clinical trial settings. A "tree-like" structure allows for in-depth investigation of behaviors that are client-specific, and results in a short interview time. Despite the sensitive nature of some questions, the interview format of the ARI-I allows subjects to comprehend all questions, and helps maintain their interest. Analyses of results show a high rate of valid responses, as characterized by a lack of inconsistent responses across similar questions. There is very little response bias. Most importantly, the scores are distributed across the entire scale.

REFERENCES

1. Edlin BR, Irwin KL, Faruque S, McCoy CB, Word C, Serrano Y, Inciardi JA, Bowser BP, Schilling RF, Holmberg SD. Intersecting epidemics–crack cocaine use and HIV infection among inner-city young adults. Multicenter Crack Cocaine and HIV Infection Study Team. N Engl J Med. 1994;331(21):1422-7.

2. Lehman JS, Allen DM, Green TA, Onorato IM. HIV infection among non-injecting drug users entering drug treatment, United States, 1989-1992. Field Services Branch. Aids. 1994;8(10):1465-9.

3. Goedert JJ, Pizza G, Gritti FM, Costigliola P, Boschini A, Bini A, Lazzari C, Palareti A. Mortality among drug users in the AIDS era. Int J Epidemiol. 1995;24(6): 1204-10.

4. Allen DM, Onorato IM, Green TA. HIV infection in intravenous drug users entering drug treatment, United States, 1988 to 1989. The Field Services Branch of the Centers for Disease Control. Am J Public Health. 1992;82(4):541-6.

5. Anonumous. HIV/AIDS Surveillance: US AIDS cases reported through December 1994. Atlanta, GA: Centers for Disease Control and Prevention; 1995.

6. Iguchi MY, Platt JJ, French JF, Baxter RC, Kushner H, Lidz VM, Bux DA, Rosen M, & Musikoff H. Correlates of HIV seropositivity among intravenous drug users not in treatment. Journal of Drug Issues. 1992;22:849-866.

7. Iguchi MY, Bux DA, Lidz V, Kushner H, French JF, Platt JJ. Interpreting HIV seroprevalence data from a street-based outreach program. J Acquir Immune Defic Syndr. 1994;7(5):491-9.

8. Bux DA, Lamb RJ, Iguchi MY. Cocaine use and HIV risk behavior in methadone maintenance patients. Drug Alcohol Depend. 1995;37(1):29-35.

9. Dwyer R, Richardson D, Ross MW, Wodak A, Miller ME, Gold J. A comparison of HIV risk between women and men who inject drugs. AIDS Educ Prev. 1994; 6(5):379-89.

10. Grella CE, Anglin MD, Wugalter SE. Cocaine and crack use and HIV risk behaviors among high-risk methadone maintenance clients. Drug Alcohol Depend. 1995;37(1):15-21.

11. Hudgins R, McCusker J, Stoddard A. Cocaine use and risky injection and sexual behaviors. Drug Alcohol Depend. 1995;37(1):7-14.

12. Iguchi MY, Bux DA, Jr., Kushner H, Lidz V, French JF, Platt JJ. Prospective evaluation of a model of risk for HIV infection among injecting drug users. Drug Alcohol Depend. 1995;40(1):63-71.

13. Joe GW, Simpson DD. HIV risks, gender, and cocaine use among opiate users. Drug Alcohol Depend. 1995;37(1):23-8.

14. Kall K. The risk of HIV infection for noninjecting sex partners of injecting drug users in Stockholm. AIDS Educ Prev. 1994;6(4):351-64.

15. Tortu S, Beardsley M, Deren S, Davis WR. The risk of HIV infection in a national sample of women with injection drug-using partners. Am J Public Health. 1994;84(8):1243-9.

16. Wodak AD, Stowe A, Ross MW, Gold J et al. HIV risk exposure of injecting drug users in Sydney. Drug & Alcohol Review. 1995;14:213-222.

17. Zapata V, Blanton C. AIDS and intravenous drug use: a growing menace. J Drug Educ. 1994;24(2):133-8.

18. Compton WM, Lamb RJ, Fletcher BW. Results of the NIDA treatment demonstration grants' cocaine workgroup: characteristics of cocaine users and HIV risk behaviors. Drug Alcohol Depend. 1995;37(1):1-6.

19. Inciardi JA, Tims FM, & Fletcher BW, ed. Innovative Approaches in the Treatment of Drug Abuse. Westport, CT: Greenwood Press; 1993.

20. Irwin KL, Edlin BR, Faruque S, McCoy HV, Word C, Serrano Y, Inciardi J, Bowser B, Holmberg SD. Crack cocaine smokers who turn to drug injection: characteristics, factors associated with injection, and implications for HIV transmission. The Multicenter Crack Cocaine and HIV Infection Study Team. Drug Alcohol Depend. 1996;42(2):85-92.

21. Greenfield L, Bigelow GE, Brooner RK. Validity of intravenous drug abusers' self-reported changes in HIV high-risk drug use behaviors. Drug Alcohol Depend. 1995;39(2):91-8.

22. Wells EA, Clark LL, Calsyn DA, Saxon AJ, Jackson TR, Wrede AF. Reporting of HIV risk behaviors by injection drug using heterosexual couples in methadone maintenance. Drug Alcohol Depend. 1994;36(1):33-8.

23. Darke S, Hall W, Heather N, Ward J, Wodak A. The reliability and validity of a scale to measure HIV risk-taking behaviour among intravenous drug users. Aids. 1991;5(2):181-5.

24. Metzger DS, DePhilippis D, Druley P, O'Brien CP, McLellan AT, Williams J, Navaline H, Dyanick S, Woody GE. The Impact of HIV Testing on Risk for AIDS Behaviors. In: Harris L, ed. College on Problems of Drug Dependence, 58th Annual Scientific Meeting; 1991:297-298.

25. Longshore D, Hsieh SC, Anglin MD. Reducing HIV risk behavior among injection drug users: effect of methadone maintenance treatment on number of sex partners. Int J Addict. 1994;29(6):741-57.

26. Morrison CS, McCusker J, Stoddard AM, Bigelow C. The validity of behavioral data reported by injection drug users on a clinical risk assessment. Int J Addict. 1995;30(7):889-99.

27. McKeganey N. Why do men buy sex and what are their assessments of the HIV-related risks when they do? AIDS Care. 1994;6(3):289-301.

28. Watters JK, Estilo MJ, Kral AH, Lorvick JJ. HIV infection among female injection-drug users recruited in community settings. Sex Transm Dis. 1994;21(6):321-8.

29. Bevier PJ, Chiasson MA, Heffernan RT, Castro KG. Women at a sexually transmitted disease clinic who reported same-sex contact: their HIV seroprevalence and risk behaviors. Am J Public Health. 1995;85(10):1366-71.

30. McQuillan GM, Khare M, Karon JM, Schable CA, Vlahov D. Update on the seroepidemiology of human immunodeficiency virus in the United States household

population: NHANES III, 1988-1994. J Acquir Immune Defic Syndr Hum Retrovirol. 1997;14(4):355-60.

31. Jacobson RL, Harris AB, Doyle MG. HIV infection and associated sexually transmitted diseases in women. Tex Med. 1995;91(3):58-60.

32. Lauver D, Armstrong K, Marks S, Schwarz S. HIV risk status and preventive behaviors among 17,619 women. J Obstet Gynecol Neonatal Nurs. 1995;24(1):33-9.

33. First MB, Spitzer RL, Gibbon M, & Williams JBW. Structured Clinical Interview for DSM-IV Axis I Disorders–patient Edition (SCID-I/O), Version 2.0.: Biometrics Research Department, New York State Psychiatric Institute; 1996.

34. Schottenfeld RS, O'Malley S, O'Connor P, & Abdul-Salaam K. Decline in intravenous drug use among treatment seeking opiate users. Journal of Substance Abuse Treatment. 1993;10:5-10.

Does Intensive
Outpatient Cocaine Treatment
Reduce AIDS Risky Behaviors?

Edward Gottheil MD, PhD
Allan Lundy, PhD
Stephen P. Weinstein, PhD
Robert C. Sterling, PhD

SUMMARY. The purposes of this study were: (1) to examine the characteristics of 447 cocaine dependent, first admission outpatients in relation to their AIDS risky behavior at intake; (2) to ascertain whether there was a reduction in risky behavior at follow-up 9 months after admission; and (3) to determine whether reductions in risky behavior were related to patient characteristics, group as compared to individual treatment, or time in treatment.

In this sample of cocaine dependent patients entering outpatient treatment, those engaging in higher AIDS risky behaviors were not

Edward Gottheil, Allan Lundy, Stephen P. Weinstein, and Robert C. Sterling are affiliated with the Department of Psychiatry and Human Behavior, Thomas Jefferson University.

Address correspondence to: Edward Gottheil MD, PhD, Department of Psychiatry and Human Behavior, Jefferson Medical College, 1201 Chestnut Street, 15th Floor, Philadelphia, PA 19107.

This research was supported in part by Grant #1 R18 DA 06166 from the National Institute on Drug Abuse and performed under the auspices of the Commonwealth Office of Drug and Alcohol Programs and the Philadelphia Department of Public Health, Coordinating Office for Drug and Alcohol Abuse Programs. Its contents are solely the responsibility of the authors and do not necessarily represent the official views of the awarding agencies NIDA, ODAP, and CODAAP.

[Haworth co-indexing entry note]: "Does Intensive Outpatient Cocaine Treatment Reduce AIDS Risky Behavior?" Gottheil, Edward et al. Co-published simultaneously in *Journal of Addictive Diseases* (The Haworth Medical Press, an imprint of The Haworth Press, Inc.) Vol. 17, No. 4, 1998, pp. 61-69; and: *Effects of Substance Abuse Treatment on AIDS Risk Behaviors* (ed: Edward Gottheil, and Barry Stimmel) The Haworth Medical Press, an imprint of The Haworth Press, Inc., 1998, pp. 61-69. Single or multiple copies of this article are available for a fee from The Haworth Document Delivery Service [1-800-342-9678, 9:00 a.m. - 5:00 p.m. (EST). E-mail address: getinfo@haworthpressinc.com].

characterized by any particular demographic profile or by a lack of knowledge about HIV/AIDS. They did have higher scores on the SCL-90-R symptom scales, the Beck Depression Inventory, and higher ratings on the Drug, Alcohol, Family, and Medical scales of the ASI.

At 9-month follow-up, AIDS risky behaviors as measured by the RAB were found to have decreased significantly. The degree of improvement was not associated with demographic variables but was predicted by higher intake problem severity and psychological symptomatology scale scores.

While improvement in risky behavior was not related to type of treatment or duration of treatment, it was related to decreased substance use. The individuals whose risky behavior decreased were those whose substance use had decreased. Improvement, then required not only being in a treatment program, but also participation and involvement in the program. Treatment and not merely attendance would seem to be critical. *[Article copies available for a fee from The Haworth Document Delivery Service: 1-800-342-9678. E-mail address: getinfo@haworthpressinc. com]*

INTRODUCTION

Substance use is clearly a major risk factor for HIV infection, and it has been hypothesized or hoped by many that substance use treatment would effectively reduce this risk.[1,2] Unfortunately, we are unable to test the hypothesis in a controlled, random assignment experiment since it would be unethical to assign these patients to treatment and no treatment conditions. As a consequence, attempts to study the effects of treatment or duration of treatment on patients' AIDS risk behaviors are confounded with the patients' motivation to enter treatment and to remain in treatment. We can, nevertheless, continue to carefully gather reliable and useful data relevant to evaluating the impact of treatment on AIDS-risk behavior.[3]

Motivation, although difficult to define or measure, must always be considered a factor involved in treatment retention, early dropout, or even the decision to contact a program in the first place. For example, in a attempt to limit the spread of HIV by increasing access to treatment for injection drug users, Sibthorpe et al.[4] offered no-cost outpatient treatment on demand to a cohort of 824 out-of-treatment injection users. Of these, 33% expressed an interest in treatment and 27% accepted a treatment coupon, but only 8% redeemed the coupon and entered treatment, and 1% remained in treatment for six months. For those deciding to enter substance abuse treatment, then, one might be more likely to expect there to be some underlying motivation to change one's behavior. Nevertheless, we found that even though 90% of a sample of 382 individuals entering outpatient substance use treatment for cocaine dependency reported having previously received AIDS information from an average of three different sources (e.g., TV, radio, newspaper, magazine, pamphlets, AIDS counseling or education, etc.) and 54% of them considered themselves at some risk for AIDS, only 40% had actually gone for testing, 26% reported having had three or more sexual partners during the last year, and 52% still had never used a condom.[5]

Moreover, while there have not been that many studies of the effect of drug treatment on AIDS risky behaviors, the results of those studies have not been entirely consistent. For opioid dependent patients in methadone maintenance treatment there is a reduction in injection drug use.[6,7] Some studies also report a reduction in the number of sexual partners and a decrease in exchanging sex for money,[8,9] but others have found no relationship between treatment and the number of sexual partners or the frequency of unprotected sex.[10,11] In a recent study, Wells et al.[12] compared individuals remaining in methadone maintenance treatment after one year who were still injecting drugs with those who had dropped out and were still injecting drugs on five factor analytic derived measures of AIDS risk behaviors. Men, but not women, retained in treatment were found to differ from those not retained on only one of the factors, i.e., less sharing of IV paraphernalia with others; women also differed on one, but a different one, of the factors, i.e., fewer drug using sexual partners.

The purpose of this study was to examine: (1) the characteristics of 447 cocaine dependent, first admission outpatients in relation to their AIDS risky behaviors at intake; (2) whether there was a reduction in risky behavior at follow-up 9 months after admission; (3) whether reductions in risky behavior were related to patient characteristics, group as compared to individual treatment, and time in treatment.

METHOD

Subjects

The subjects of this study were individuals who had volunteered for a larger investigation involving a randomized controlled trial comparing individual counseling and intensive outpatient treatments.[13] They were 447 patients recruited from among first admissions to our Intensive Outpatient Cocaine Treatment Clinic; at least 18 years of age, with a DSM-III-R diagnosis of cocaine dependence who were not overtly psychotic, actively suicidal or so cognitively impaired as to be unable to understand informed consent or to participate in our programming.

Assessments

Intake information included: (a) brief intake form covering basic demographic data, previous treatment and employment histories, and personal and family history of substance use; (b) self-administered Milcom, a health questionnaire providing personal and family medical history and medical review of systems;[14] (c) urine drug screen; (d) Risky AIDS Behavior Inventory (RAB) which gives equal weight to and combines items relating to needle risk, i.e., injected drugs, shared works, visited shooting gallery, used new needles, cleaned needle and works, how cleaned, and items relating to sex risk, i.e., number of different sex partners in the past six months and frequency of condom use when having sex in the past six months;[15] (e) Addiction Severity Index (ASI) indicating difficulties in seven problem areas;[16] (f) Beck Depression Inventory;[17] and (g) SCL-90-R Symptom Checklist,[18] a quick, multifactor measure of global psychopathology. Instruments not administered during the first intake visit, due in large part to the time of day the patient arrived at the clinic, were usually given during a second visit to the program at which time an AIDS Knowledge Survey (AKS) was also administered, an AIDS educational module presented and the AKS administered again. Since 88 (19.7%) of the 447 patients did not return for a second visit, the number of cases available for analysis varied from measure to measure.

Treatment

According to the design of the larger study (13), patients were randomly assigned to 12 weeks of either outpatient individual counseling one hour per week (IND), one hour per week of individual plus a one-hour weekly group (IND-GRP), or to therapeutic and activity groups for three hours, three times a week (INT). Follow-up interviews were scheduled at nine months following admission and were conducted by an independent contractor. The follow-up consisted of phone administration of the ASI and RAB as well as some discussion about how the individual was adjusting since leaving the treatment program.

RESULTS

The participants in the study were 61.3% male, 93.5% African-American and averaged 31.9 years of age and 11.4 years of schooling. They were 90.6% unemployed and 75.6% had never married. Regarding cocaine use, they met DSM-III-R criteria and were judged to exhibit an average of 7.2 of the nine DSM-III-R substance use dependence criteria. They reported having used for an average of 7.0 years and on 7.8 of the last 30 days. Urinalyses on admission were positive for cocaine in 51.6%. The average ASI drug severity score was 6.3 and the number of prior drug treatments was 1.1. When there was a second drug (59.3), it was most commonly alcohol (77.4%). Of the 447 patients, 88 (19.7%) did not return for a second visit. The dropouts did not differ from those who returned on demographic variables such as age, sex, race, marital status, employment, income, legal difficulties, years of drug use or prior drug treatment history. They did differ on education, 11.09 ± 1.74 yrs as compared to 11.49 ± 1.70 yrs for those who returned (t = 2.03, 445df p < .05). Education, however, was not related to admission RAB scores or to change in RAB scores from admission to follow-up.

AIDS risky behavior as measured by the RAB was not found to be correlated significantly with intake variables such as age, sex, race, education, marital status, employment, income, prior treatment, previous misdemeanors or felonies, AIDS knowledge, or the number of DSM-III-R criteria for Cocaine Dependence rated as present. The reported frequency of cocaine use in the last month was related to the RAB (r = .11, p < .05), as was years of use (r = .11, p < .05), but presence of cocaine in the intake urinalysis was not.

Since not all of the instruments were administered to all of the patients, the correlations of the ASI, BDI and SCL-90 scales with the RAB, as reported in Table 1, are based on different numbers of available cases. High scores on the RAB were found to be associated with problem severity on the Medical (r = .12, p < .05), Alcohol (r = .15, p < .01), Drug (r = .19, p < .001), and Family (r = .15, p < .01) scales of the ASI, the BDI (r .= 11, p < .05), and on most of the SCL-90-R symptom scales including the overall GSI (r = .18, p < .001), PSI (r = .13, p < .05), and PST (r = .18, p < .01) scales. Interestingly, patients with high RAB scores remained longer in treatment (r = .15, p < .01) than those characterized by less risky behaviors.

At follow-up, nine months after admission, 316 (70.7%) of the 447 patients were located and completed follow-up interviews. For those individuals for whom we had both intake and follow-up data, the intake mean RAB score of 8.52 ± 4.86 was found to be significantly decreased to 7.67 ± 4.49 (t = 2.81, df = 284, p < .05). Degree of improvement from intake to follow-up was not found to be associated with age, sex, race, education, marital status, employment, income, years of use, prior treatment, previous misdemeanors or felonies, or knowledge about AIDS. Those individuals who from intake to follow-up decreased their risk taking behaviors, however, were those who at intake had higher ASI alcohol (r = .14, p < .05), drug (r = .16, p < .05) and legal (r = .16, p < .05) problem severity scores and elevated symptomatology scores on the Obsessive-Compulsive (r = .13, p < 05), Interpersonal Sensitivity (r = .14, p < 05), GSI (r = .14, p < .05) and PSI (r = .16, p < .05) measures of the SCL-90 (Table 1).

No differences were found in improvement for AIDS risky behaviors according to treatment group, i.e., individual, individual plus group, or intensive treatment (F = .63, df = 2, 282, p > .05). Furthermore, even though there was a decrease in RAB scores from intake to follow-up, the decrease in risky

TABLE 1. Correlations Between Intake Variables and (A) Intake RAB Scores and (B) Change in RAB Scores from Intake to Follow-Up.

	Intake RAB	RAB Change
Addiction Severity Index:	N = 339	N = 234
Medical	.12*	.11
Employment	− .04	.05
Alcohol	.15**	.14*
Drug	.19**	.16*
Legal	.05	.16*
Family/Social	.15**	.09
Psychological	.05	.09
Beck Depression Index	N = 405	N = 280
	.11*	.11
SCL-90	N = 398	N = 277
Somatization	.13**	.09
Obsessive-Compulsive	.17***	.13*
Interpersonal Sensitivity	.20***	.14*
Depression	.16**	.12
Anxiety	.16**	.12
Hostility	.10	.09
Phobic Anxiety	.09	.03
Paranoid Ideation	.10	.04
Psychoticism	.14**	.10
Global Severity Index	.18***	.14*
Positive Symptom Index	.13**	.16**
Positive Symptom Total	.18***	.10

*p < .05,   2-tailed
**p < .01,   2-tailed
***p < .001,   2-tailed

behaviors was not found to be related to time in treatment (r = .09, n = 285 p > .05) and comparing those individuals, for example, who remained in the program six weeks or longer with those who left prior to six weeks, we found no difference whatsoever in RAB scores at nine-month follow-up. We might also note that in the randomized controlled trial no differences among the treatment groups were found with respect to either retention or the number of early dropouts.[13]

RAB total scores at follow-up, however, were related (Table 2) to follow-up scores on the ASI drug composite (r = .21, p < .001), the ASI alcohol composite (r = .23, p < .001), and the number of days of cocaine use in the last 30 days (r = .18, p < .01). Moreover, improvement from intake to follow-up in RAB scores was related to improvement in ASI drug (r = .20, p < .01) and alcohol (r = .29, p < .001) scores and to a decrease in the number of days

TABLE 2. Correlations Between Substance Use and Risky AIDS Behaviors for (A) Follow-Up Scores and (B) Change from Intake to Follow-Up Scores.

	N	Sex Risk	Needle Risk	Total Risk
Follow-Up:				
ASI Drug	300	.16**	.23***	.21***
ASI Alc	297	.19***	.16**	.23***
Days COC/30	302	.15*	.14*	.18**
Improvement:				
ASI Drug	197	.16*	.11	.20**
ASI Alc	197	.26***	.14*	.29***
Days COC/30	238	.18**	.11*	.21***

*p < .05,   2-tailed
**p < .01,   2-tailed
***p < .001,   2-tailed

of cocaine use in the previous 30 days (r = .21, p < .001). Thus individuals whose risky behaviors decreased were those whose substance use had decreased.

DISCUSSION

In this sample of 447 individuals entering an outpatient treatment program for cocaine dependency, those engaging in higher AIDS risky behaviors were not characterized by any particular demographic profile or by a lack of knowledge about AIDS. They did, however, have higher scores on most of the SCL-90-R symptom scales and higher ratings on the Drug, Alcohol, Family, and Medical scales of the ASI. Possibly related to their psychological profile and multiple problem severity, they also remained longer in treatment.

At nine-month follow-up, AIDS risky behaviors as measured by the RAB were found to have decreased significantly. The degree of improvement was not associated with demographic variables but was related to higher problem severity and psychological symptomatology scale scores at intake. Starting off with higher scores and presumably greater distress, they may have had more room to improve and more interest in remaining in treatment and doing so.

Improvement was not found to be related to neither the type of treatment (Individual, Individual plus Group, Intensive) nor the duration of treatment. Although RAB scores decreased significantly from the time of treatment entry to follow-up and those with higher RAB scores at entry remained longer in treatment, the decrease in scores was not related to time spent in treatment. It should be noted that the findings are subject to the limitations of a telephone follow-up procedure and a 70% follow-up rate as well as our particular treatment methodology and study variables. The decrease we found in RAB scores, however, was found to be associated with decreased substance use. Individuals whose risky behaviors decreased were those whose substance use had decreased.

Retention in substance abuse treatment alone was not sufficient for improvement in risky behaviors to occur. Patients may remain in a treatment program for a variety of reasons without really participating. Some may not improve and some may become worse. To decrease AIDS risky behaviors, then, requires not merely entering into a substance abuse treatment program but also participating in and profiting from the program as indicated, for example, by improvement in other respects such as decreased drug use. Treatment and not merely attendance would seem to be the critical variable.

REFERENCES

1. Centers for Disease Control. HIV/AIDS surveillance report. Atlanta: Centers for Disease Control, April 1992.

2. Bracken PAW, Toreros RCA, Barrens M, et al. Recommendations for control and prevention of human immunodeficiency virus (HIV) infection in intravenous drug users. Ann. Int. Med. 1989:110:833-837.

3. Gottheil E, McLella AT, and Druley KA. Reasonable and unreasonable methodological standards for the evaluation of alcoholism treatment. In E. Gottheil, McLellan AT, and Druley KA (eds). Matching Patient Needs and Treatment Methods in Alcoholism and Drug Abuse. Springfield, IL: Charles C Thomas. 1981:371-389.

4. Sibthorpe B, Fleming D, Tesselaar H, Gould J, and Nichols L. The response of injection drug users to free treatment on demand: implications for HIV control. Am. J. Drug Alcohol Abuse. 1996:22:203-215.

5. Gottheil E, Weinstein SP, Sterling RC. Acceptance of HIV testing by substance-abusing individuals. Am J. Addictions. 1993:2:212-219.

6. Williams AB, McNelly EA, Williams AE, and D'Aguila RT. Methadone maintenance treatment and HIV type 1 seroconversion among injecting drug users. AIDS Care. 1992:4:35-41.

7. Longshore D, Hsieh S, Danila B, and Anglin MD. Methadone maintenance and needle/syringe sharing. Int. J. Addict. 1993:28:983-996.

8. Longshore D, Hsieh S, and Anglin MD. Reducing HIV risk behavior among injection drug users: Effect of methadone maintenance treatment on number of sex partners. Int. J. Addict. 1994:29:741-757.

9. Watkins RE, Metzger D, Woody GE, and McLellan AT. High-risk sexual behaviors of intravenous drug users in- and out-of-treatment: Implications for the spread off infection. Am. J. Drug Alcohol Abuse. 1992:18:389-398.

10. Abdul-Quader AS, Friedman SR, Des Jarlals D, Marmor MM, Maslansky R, and Bartelme S. Methadone maintenance and behavior by intravenous drug users that can transmit HIV. Contemp. Drug Prob. 1988:14:424-434.

11. Neaigus S, Sufian M, Friedman SR, Goldsmith D, Stepherson B, Mota P, Pascal J, and DesJarlais DC. Effects of outreach intervention risk reduction among intravenous drug users. AIDS Educ. Prevent. 1990:2:253-271.

12. Wells EA, Calsyn DA, Clark LL, Saxon AJ, and Jackson TR. Retention in methadone maintenance is associated with reductions in different HIV risk behaviors for women and men. Am. J. Drug Alcohol Abuse. 1996:22:509-523.

13. Weinstein SP, Gottheil E, and Sterling RC. Randomized comparison of intensive outpatient vs. individual therapy for cocaine abusers. Journal of Addictive Diseases. 1997:165(2):41-56.

14. Milcom Systems. Milcom. Libertyville, IL: Milcom Systems, Hollister Inc. 1989.

15. Metzger DS, Woody GE, DePhillipis D, McLella AT, O'Brien CP, and Platt JJ. Risk factors for needle sharing among methadone-treated patients. Am. J. Psychiatry. 1991:148:636-640.

16. McLellan AT, Luborsky L, Cacciola J, Griffith J, and Evans F. New data from the Addiction Severity Index: Reliability and validity in three centers. J. Nerv. Ment. Dis. 1985:173:412-423.

17. Beck AT. Cognitive Therapy and the Emotional Disorders. New York, NY: International Universities Press. 1976.

18. Derogatis LR. SCL-90-R: Administration, Scoring, and Procedures Manual-II. Towson, MD: Clinical Psychometrics. 1983.

Changes in HIV Risk Behaviors Among Cocaine-Using Methadone Patients

Stephen Magura, PhD
Andrew Rosenblum, PhD
Eric M. Rodriguez, MA

SUMMARY. Cocaine use among methadone patients has been related to higher prevalence of HIV risk behaviors. HIV risk behaviors for cocaine-using patients in methadone treatment (N = 207) were examined for two time periods, the current month in-treatment and the month previous to treatment admission. All needle-related and sexually-related risk behaviors (except for needle hygiene) significantly and substantially declined over the average two year time interval. Several variables were associated with needle and sexual risks in multivariate regression analyses. Dropping apparent opiate use underreporters from the analyses did not alter the results. From a harm reduction perspective, high priority should be given to retaining cocaine-using patients in methadone maintenance, intensifying in-program services for those with anti-

---

Stephen Magura, Andrew Rosenblum, and Eric M. Rodriguez are affiliated with National Development and Research Institutes, 2 World Trade Center, New York, NY 10048.

This study was conducted in collaboration with the Narcotics Rehabilitation Center (NRC), Mt. Sinai Medical Center, New York, NY (Barry Stimmel, MD, Executive Director). Funded by Grant No. 5 R18 DA06959 from the National Institute on Drug Abuse. Thanks are extended to Sy Demsky, Administrator; Victor Sturiano, Clinical Director; Philip Parris, Clinic Physician; and the entire staff of the NRC for their contributions to the conduct of the study. Preliminary results were presented at the American Society of Addiction Medicine Annual Conference, San Diego, CA, April, 1997.

[Haworth co-indexing entry note]: "Changes in HIV Risk Behaviors Among Cocaine-Using Methadone Patients." Magura, Stephen, Andrew Rosenblum, and Eric M. Rodriguez. Co-published simultaneously in *Journal of Addictive Diseases* (The Haworth Medical Press, an imprint of The Haworth Press, Inc.) Vol. 17, No. 4, 1998, pp. 71-90; and: *Effects of Substance Abuse Treatment on AIDS Risk Behaviors* (ed: Edward Gottheil, and Barry Stimmel) The Haworth Medical Press, an imprint of The Haworth Press, Inc., 1998, pp. 71-90. Single or multiple copies of this article are available for a fee from The Haworth Document Delivery Service [1-800-342-9678, 9:00 a.m. - 5:00 p.m. (EST). E-mail address: getinfo@haworthpressinc.com].

social personality, bipolar disorder or alcoholism, as well as increasing access to needle exchanges and free condoms. *[Article copies available for a fee from The Haworth Document Delivery Service: 1-800-342-9678. E-mail address: getinfo@haworthpressinc.com]*

INTRODUCTION

The effectiveness of methadone maintenance in reducing heroin use and illegal activities and in increasing pro-social behaviors has been demonstrated.[1-4] Methadone treatment has assumed particular importance in view of the HIV epidemic among drug injectors that began in the early 1980's. Most heroin users historically have been drug injectors; thus reductions in heroin use and drug injection (and often, equipment sharing) have occurred concomitantly among those entering methadone treatment.[5-12] Methadone treatment has also been associated with reduction of sexually related HIV risk behaviors.[11,13-15] The effect of methadone treatment on reducing HIV transmission is indicated by the substantially lower HIV seroprevalence rates usually associated with being enrolled in treatment and with longer time in treatment.[16-21]

Many entrants to methadone treatment are dually addicted to heroin and cocaine, which may involve simultaneous injection of heroin and cocaine ("speedballing"), inhalation (smoking "crack" or "rock") or intranasal use ("sniffing").[22-25] Among injectors, cocaine injection is associated with more frequent injection[26] and higher HIV seroprevalence.[27] A study of IDUs in nine San Francisco methadone programs found that daily cocaine injection significantly increased the rate of HIV infection as compared with heroin injection only.[18] Similarly, frequency of cocaine injection was the strongest correlate of HIV seropositivity in a methadone treatment sample.[28]

Specifically, methadone patients who continue (or begin) to use cocaine during treatment have more frequent and severe HIV risk behaviors than those not using cocaine. Cocaine and non-cocaine users in methadone maintenance were compared on HIV risk behaviors for the previous month.[29] The patients were volunteers from five clinics in the greater Philadelphia area who had been enrolled for a mean of 36 months. Cocaine users were more likely to inject drugs and had greater frequencies of injections and sexual contacts without condoms; this was independent of heroin and other drug use, time in treatment, age, gender and minority status. No differences were found in frequency of injections with shared equipment (likely due to large variances on this measure), number of people with whom equipment was shared, and number of sex partners. The study suggests that cocaine use among methadone patients maintains injecting behavior (85% of cocaine users inject) but its effect on needle sharing is unclear.

A study of methadone patients in Sidney found that, among patients who injected in the previous month, those who injected cocaine had a higher level of injection risk (more frequent, more sharing) than patients injecting only other drugs. However, cocaine users and non-users were similar on sexual risk-taking.[30] In contrast, another study reported that cocaine use was significantly related to all measures of injection and sex-related HIV risk behaviors.[11]

This prior research has shown that methadone patients who use cocaine are at higher HIV risk than those not using cocaine. However, it is possible that even patients who continue cocaine use during treatment may have reduced their HIV risk behaviors, although perhaps less than those who never used or stopped using cocaine during treatment. This requires a longitudinal perspective, i.e., comparing pre-treatment with during-treatment HIV risk behaviors.

Only one longitudinal study has examined changes in HIV risks among methadone patients who use cocaine. The study selected new Texas methadone admissions who were injectors and remained in treatment at least six months; their HIV behaviors were assessed from intake to months 3 and 6 of treatment.[11] At intake, cocaine users were more likely to share injection equipment and have more sex partners than non-users. However, risk reduction for cocaine users and non-users was similar in magnitude over the six month interval for all risk variables examined: injection, sharing injection equipment, multiple sex partners and unprotected sex. HIV risks also were reduced for patients who continued to inject drugs during treatment.

The current study extends previous research on HIV risk reduction during methadone treatment in several ways. First, it focuses on changes within the highest HIV risk group in methadone programs, those currently dependent on cocaine/crack, in order to confirm the behavior changes reported by previous research.[11] This study will examine methadone treatment's utility for harm reduction even among the most problematic patients and could lead to a reappraisal of treatment and discharge policies for such patients. Second, in contrast to previous research, this study has made available a wider range of possible predictors of risk behaviors including lifetime and current DSM diagnoses. Third, the study patients had been in treatment for varying lengths of time, allowing time in treatment to be included as a predictor of HIV risk reduction. Lastly, unlike the previous research cited above, this study will address the accuracy of patients' reports of drug use.

METHODS

Subjects: Patients in a methadone maintenance program in Manhattan (about 700 slots) who entered a clinical research trial that tested several supplementary therapies for cocaine dependence/abuse (N = 207). Study intake was during 1991-1994. (Description of the clinical trial is given in a previous paper.[31])

Inclusion Criteria: (1) Lifetime DSM-III-R diagnosis of opiate dependence and current diagnosis of cocaine dependence or abuse. (2) At least one-cocaine positive urine in the four weeks prior to recruitment. (3) Receiving the same daily dose of methadone for at least one month.

Exclusion Criteria: Failing a psychotic screen (4.5% of screened patients failed).

Procedures: Participation was voluntary with informed consent; an incentive of $25 was given for completing the interview protocol. Data collection included a study-developed psychosocial history interview, the Structured Clinical Interview (SCID) for DSM-III-R[32] and the Brief Symptom Inventory (BSI).[33] The interviews were conducted by experienced research staff with masters (3) and bachelors (1) degrees who received formal training in SCID administration by qualified trainers. All SCID diagnoses were reviewed and confirmed by a psychiatrist or licensed clinical psychologist. Clinic urinalysis data were obtained, consisting of weekly enzyme immunoassays for opiates, cocaine, benzodiazepines, barbiturates and methadone.

Design of Current Study: Patients were interviewed and diagnosed before receiving any study cocaine therapies. The analytical design is retrospective: patients were queried about HIV risk behaviors for the last 30 days (termed "in-treatment") and for the 30 day period prior to their methadone clinic admission, which was an average of about 2 years ago (termed "pre-treatment"). Comparisons of HIV risk behaviors will be between these two periods of time.

Measures

Needle-Related HIV Risks

- Injection Frequency (Number of injections per week)
- Needle Sharing Risk (Composite of seven questions: how often rent works, borrow needle/set, use same cooker, use works after someone, use works before someone, share drugs, use a house needle/set? Responses: all, most, half, some of the time; 1-2 times only; never)
- Needle Hygiene Risk (Composite of six questions: how often rinse with bleach, rinse with alcohol, boil in water, rinse with hot water, rinse with cold water, wipe with alcohol swab? Same responses as above)
- Own Works Used (How often? Same responses as above)
- Needle Risk Composite (Composite of Injection Frequency and Needle Sharing Risk)

Sexually-Related HIV Risks

- Multiple Partners (Number of sexual partners)
- Drug Risk Sexual Partners (Composite of three items: numbers of drug injecting, other drug-using and needle-sharing partners)
- Sex Exchange Risk Partners (Composite of four items: how often gave or got money for sex; how often gave or got drugs for sex. Responses: 5-7, 2-4, 1 day[s] a week; 1-2 times only; never)
- Unprotected Sex (How often used condoms for sex. Responses: all, most, half, some of the time; 1-2 times only; never)
- Sexual Partner Risk Composite (Composite of Multiple Partners, Drug Risk Sex Partners, Sex Exchange Risk Partners)

Predictor Variables

These were selected for inclusion because previous studies have found variables in these domains (sociodemographics, treatment history, psychiatric diagnosis and severity, substance use and criminal activity) to be related to HIV risk behaviors and/or seropositivity

- Gender
- Race/Ethnicity (Hispanic, African-American, White/Other)
- Age (years)
- Education (years)
- Living Arrangement Stability (homeless, someone else's home/apartment, own home/apartment)
- Employment (on or off the books in last 30 days; yes or no)
- Prior Treatment Admissions (total number of drug abuse treatment or detoxification programs)
- Time in Methadone Treatment (this episode)
- Methadone Dosage (daily mg at interview time)
- DSM-III-R Disorders
  - Lifetime and Current Bipolar
  - Lifetime and Current Major Depression
  - Lifetime and Current Mood (any)
  - Lifetime and Current Anxiety
  - Anti-Social Personality (ASPD)
- HIV Status (reported positive vs. other; reported negative vs. other)
- Heroin Frequency (number of days used in last 30)
- Cocaine Frequency (number of days used in last 30)
- Heavy Alcohol Use (number of days in last 30 with 4 or more drinks/day)
- Brief Symptom Inventory (Global Severity Index)

- Property Offenses (yes or no in last 30 days, by self-report)
- Violent Offenses (yes or no in last 30 days, by self-report)
- Drug Sales Offenses (excluding possession; yes or no in last 30 days, by self-report)

Analytical Methods

Changes in HIV risk behaviors are assessed in two ways: crosstabulating pre- and in-treatment risk behavior categories and computing paired t-tests of risk variables for the two time periods. Changes in risk behaviors are assessed for the entire sample as well as for certain subsets of patients at risk while in-treatment, i.e., those who continued to inject drugs and those who continued both to inject and share needles.

Multiple regression analyses are conducted to determine predictors of change in risk behavior after entering treatment. For the multiple regressions, all predictor variables which correlated at the $p = .10$ significance level with the given dependent variable, along with the pre-treatment measure of the dependent variable, were entered into a backwards elimination procedure. Analysis of residuals was conducted; all analyses reported conform to the requirements of linearity and homogeneity of variances. Cases were excluded as necessary to eliminate or minimize the number of statistical outliers. All statistical procedures were performed with SPSS.[34]

RESULTS

Background Characteristics

Table 1 presents background characteristics of the sample at the in-treatment interview time. Females were purposely oversampled by the study; about 70% are male in the program as a whole. The sample is about one-half Hispanic because the program is located in East Harlem, a predominantly Hispanic community. About one-third were single, about two-thirds had a high school or equivalency degree and about one-fifth were employed full time; few (6%) could be characterized as homeless. The sample had a mean of seven previous treatment (any type) and detoxification episodes and a mean time in treatment for this episode of 28 months. Frequency of heroin use was relatively low, occurring on an average of three days in the last 30 days; 58% reported no heroin use during that period; and 50% had all urines negative for opiates during that period. Frequency of cocaine use was high, occurring on an average of 20 days in the last 30 days, with 35% reporting use every day. Heavy alcohol use was also relatively low, occurring on four

TABLE 1. Sample Description (N = 207)

Gender	
Male	59%
Race/Ethnicity	
Hispanic	53%
African-American	36
White	11
Age (mean, s.d.)	38.5 years (7.5)
Marital Status	
Single	36%
Married	32
Divorced/Separated	32
Living Arrangements	
Own home/apartment	84%
Someone else's home/apartment	10
Homeless	6
Education	
Less than high school	30%
High school/GED	48
Some college	22
Employed (full-time)	18%
Prior Treatment Detox/Admissions (mean, s.d.)	7.0 (5.8)
Time in Treatment (mean, s.d.)	27.8 months (37.6)
Methadone Dosage (mean, s.d.)	67mg (18)
Heroin Frequency (days in last 30)	3.2 (6.2)
Cocaine Frequency (days in last 30)	19.6 (10.0)
Heavy Alcohol Use (days in last 30)	3.7 (8.1)
HIV Status	
Positive	24%
Negative	45
Unknown/Untested/Not reported	31
DSM-III-R Disorders (current)	
Major Depression	29%
Bipolar	5
Mood (any)	40
Anxiety (any)	29
Anti-Social Personality (ASPD)	25
Brief Symptom Inventory-GSI (mean, s.d.)	1.08 (.77)
Drug Sales Offenses (last 30 days)	24%
Property Offenses (last 30 days)	16%
Violent Offenses (last 30 days)	3%

days out of 30, with 68% reporting no days of heavy alcohol use. One-quarter reported being HIV seropositive; the proportion in the entire sample might be higher, if we assume that some in the "unknown/untested/not reported" category are seropositive as well.

Psychiatric co-morbidity is high, similar to the findings of previous research in methadone populations (for a review see Magura et al.[35]). The mean BSI-GSI score (1.08) is closer to the mean of psychiatric outpatients (1.32) than to that of non-patient normals (.30).[36]

The most prevalent criminal activity is drug sales-related, with about one-quarter reporting that for the last month. Property offenses (mainly shoplifting) were reported by 16% and violent offenses by very few (3%).

Shifts in HIV Risk Behaviors–Categorical Analysis

Table 2 indicates the types of shifts in drug injection and paraphernalia sharing activities between the last month pre-treatment and the current month in-treatment. Among those with no injection pre-treatment, very few (4%) had shifted to injecting in-treatment. Among those injecting, but not sharing pre-treatment, one-half had shifted to no injection in-treatment. Among those injecting and sharing pre-treatment, about one-third had shifted to no injection and about one-fifth shifted to injection without sharing.

Table 3 indicates the types of shifts in sexual partner risks between pre-treatment and in-treatment. Among those reporting no sexual partners at pre-treatment, 16% reported at least one sexual partner (but without specific risk characteristics) and an additional 16% reported at least one high risk partner. Among those with low risk partners at pre-treatment, about one-half reported no sexual partner and about one fifth reported at least one high risk

TABLE 2. Shifts in Injection and Sharing

Pre-Treatment: No Injection			
In-Treatment:	No Injection 96%	Inject, No Share 3%	Inject & Share 1%	(N) 77

Pre–Treatment: Injecting, No Sharing			
In-Treatment:	No Injection 50%	Inject, No Share 47%	Inject & Share 3%	(N) 30

Pre-Treatment: Injecting and Sharing			
In-Treatment:	No Injection 37%	Inject, No Share 19%	Inject & Share 44%	(N) 100

TABLE 3. Shifts in Sexual Partner Risks

Pre-Treatment: No Sex Partners			
In-Treatment:	No Sex	Low Risk	High Risk	(N)
	68%	16%	16%	50

Pre-Treatment: Low Risk Partners[1]			
In-Treatment:	No Sex	Low Risk	High Risk	(N)
	51%	30%	19%	37

Pre-Treatment: High Risk Partners[2]			
In-Treatment:	No Sex	Low Risk	High Risk	(N)
	22%	12%	66%	130

1. No specific risks related to drug use or sex exchanges.
2. Drug-using and/or sex exchange partners.

partner at in-treatment. Among those with high risk partners at pre-treatment, one-third reported either no sex or low risk partners only at in-treatment.

Table 4 indicates the types of shifts in unprotected sex (i.e., no condom use) between pre-treatment and in-treatment. Among those with no sex partners at pre-treatment, but who report sex at in-treatment, about two-thirds use condoms inconsistently. Among those always using condoms during sex at pre-treatment (only 14% of the sample), small but about equal numbers shifted to either no sex or using condoms inconsistently at in-treatment. Finally, among those using condoms inconsistently for sex at pre-treatment, about one-third shifted to no sex and about one-tenth to consistent condom use at in-treatment.

Changes in HIV Risk Behaviors–Parametric Analysis

Table 5 shows the results of paired t-tests comparing specific needle-related HIV risk behaviors between pre-treatment and in-treatment. Some of the analyses are conducted for the entire sample and some for subgroups–in-treatment injectors only or in-treatment sharers only. The subgroup analyses are intended to determine whether the *degree* of risk behavior has changed even for those patients who continue to engage in specific risk behaviors in-treatment. All needle-related risk behaviors significantly and substantially declined for each comparison except one: needle hygiene (i.e., cleaning) risks for the small number of in-treatment needle sharers did not change.

Table 6 shows the results of paired t-tests comparing specific sexually-related HIV risk behaviors between pre-treatment and in-treatment; all measures show statistically significant reductions. Some of the risk reduction is

TABLE 4. Shifts in Unprotected Sex

Pre-Treatment: No Sex Partners			
In-Treatment:	No Sex 70%	Condoms Always 10%	Inconsistent 20%	(N) 49

Pre-Treatment: Condoms, Always Use			
In-Treatment:	No Sex 14%	Condoms Always 75%	Inconsistent 11%	(N) 28

Pre-Treatment: Condoms, Inconsistent Use			
In-Treatment:	No Sex 32%	Condoms Always 13%	Inconsistent 55%	(N) 122

TABLE 5. Changes in Needle-Related HIV Risks

Variable	Pre-Tx Mean	S.D.	In-Tx Mean	S.D.	(t, df)	Paired 2-tailed Sig.
Heroin Frequency	27.85	(6.49)	3.23	(6.20)	(40.83, 205)	.000
Injection Frequency	17.64	(27.42)	4.45	(16.92)	(6.24, 205)	.000
Injection Frequency (for In-Treatment Injectors)	32.72	(35.71)	11.45	(25.73)	(4.27, 79)	.000
Needle Sharing Risk (for In-Treatment Injectors)	7.49	(6.87)	3.70	(5.07)	(4.88, 76)	.000
Own Works Used (for In-Treatment Injectors)	3.23	(1.23)	3.71	(.81)	(−3.74, 72)	.000
Needle Hygiene Risk (for In-Treatment Sharers)	6.28	(4.98)	6.45	(5.06)	(−0.32, 28)	N.S.
Needle Risk Composite	9.57	(10.82)	2.52	(5.48)	(9.94, 203)	.000
Needle Risk Composite (for In-Treatment Injectors)	15.96	(9.74)	6.58	(7.21)	(7.73, 77)	.000

TABLE 6. Changes in Sexually-Related HIV Risks

Variable	Pre-Tx Mean	S.D.	In-Tx Mean	S.D.	(t, df)	Paired 2-tailed Sig
Number of Partners	3.77	(15.78)	1.64	(4.91)	(2.60, 202)	.01
Number of Partners (Sexually Active at In-Treatment)	5.16	(19.81)	2.60	(6.00)	(1.95, 126)	.05
Drug Risk Partners (Sexually Active at In–Treatment)	1.83	(4.03)	1.17	(2.93)	(2.16, 122)	.03
Sex Exchange Partners (Sexually Active at In-Treatment)	.98	(2.13)	.48	(1.47)	(3.21, 123)	.002
Sexual Partner Risk Composite	.21	(.20)	.12	(.15)	(7.09, 206)	.000
Sexual Partner Risk Composite (Sexually Active at In-Treatment)	.25	(.21)	.19	(.15)	(3.64, 129)	.000
Unprotected Sex (Sexually Active at In-Treatment)	3.03	(2.30)	2.53	(2.08)	(2.99, 121)	.003

attributable to a decrease of those with a sex partner (compare Table 3), but even for those sexually active at in-treatment, numbers of drug-using and sex exchange risk partners decline as well. Unprotected sex decreases slightly but significantly on the 6-point scale of condom use.

Predictors of Changes in HIV Risk–Multivariate Analysis

Multiple regressions using backward elimination of predictor variables that had been significant at $p = .10$ were performed for five HIV risk variables that represent the range of major risk behaviors: injection frequency, needle sharing risk, needle risk composite, sexual partner risk composite and unprotected sex. (Specifically, length of time in treatment at the interview time was not associated with any risk behaviors in preliminary bivariate analysis. Methadone dosage at the interview time was associated only with the needle risk composite, such that higher dose was associated with higher risk [$r = .16$, $p < .05$].)

Table 7 presents the results for the needle risk variables. The sexually-related HIV risk variables were candidates as covariates, because of possible links between needle risks and sexual partner risks. Three factors were associated with injection frequency at in-treatment: heroin use frequency, current bipolar disorder and anti-social personality disorder. Four factors were associated with needle-sharing risk at in-treatment–cocaine use frequency, violent offenses, being HIV-positive and being female. Factors associated with needle risk, a composite of injection and needle-sharing frequencies, were:

TABLE 7. Multiple Regression-Needle Risk at In-Treatment (Backward Elimination)

	Dependent Variables					
	Injection Frequency[2]		Needle Sharing Risk[3]		Needle Risk Composite[4]	
Predictors[1]	Beta	Sig t	Beta	Sig t	Beta	Sig t
Heroin Frequency	.48	.000	a		.43	.000
Cocaine Frequency	b		.18	.05	b	
Bipolar-Current	.22	.001	a		.17	.005
Anti-Social Personality	.13	.04	a		b	
Violent Offenses	a		.44	.000	.20	.001
HIV-Positive	a		.27	.006	b	
Gender-Female	a		.33	.001	a	
Needle Risk Composite Pre-Treatment)	a		a		.17	.000
	$R^2 = .31$ (N = 183)		$R^2 = .40$ (N = 77)		$R^2 = .42$ (N = 177)	

a. Did not qualify for inclusion in initial regression.

b. Included in initial regression, excluded by backward elimination

1. All predictors measured at in-treatment useless otherwise specified.

2. Other covariates in the initial regression were: Injection Frequency (pre-tx), Living Arrangement Stability.

3. Other covariates in the initial regression were: Needle Sharing Risk (pre-tx), Heavy Alcohol Use, Drug Risk Sex Partners (excluding needle-sharing partners). Included only subjects who injected at pre-treatment or in-treatment.

4. Other covariates in the initial regression were: Property Offenses, Prior Treatment Admissions, Multiple Partners, Living Arrangement Stability, Methadone Dosage, Drug Risk Sex Partners (excluding needle-sharing partners).

heroin use frequency, current bipolar disorder, violent offenses, and needle risk score at pre-treatment. (Methadone dose lost significance in this multivariate analysis.)

Table 8 presents the regression results for the sexually-related HIV risk variables. There was a strong association between being white and being diagnosed with anti-social personality disorder (both of which were signifi-

TABLE 8. Multiple Regression–Sexual HIV Risk at In-Treatment (Backward Elimination)

	Dependent Variables			
	Sexual Partner Risk Composite[2]		Unprotected Sex[3]	
Predictors[1]	Beta	Sig t	Beta	Sig t
Total Treatment Admissions	.15	.006	a	
Drug Sales Offenses	.09	.09	−.16	.01
Heavy Alcohol Use	.16	.004	a	
ASPD X White	.29	.000	a	
Gender-Female	a		.14	.03
Education	a		−.19	.004
Drug Risk Sex Partners[4]	a		−.18	.008
Sex Partner Risk Composite (Pre-Treatment)	.48	.000	b	
Unprotected Sex (Pre-Treatment, latest sexually active month)	a		.56	.000
	R^2 = .48 (N = 182)		R^2 = .51 (N = 123)	

a. Didn't qualify for inclusion in initial regression.
b. Included in initial regression, excluded by backward elimination
1. All predictors measured at in-treatment unless otherwise specified.
2. High score = high number of partners and risk partners. Other covariates in the initial regression were: ASPD, Race-White, Cocaine Frequency, Major Depression.
3. Highest score = never use condoms. Lowest score = always use condoms. Other covariates in the initial regression were: HIV- Positive, Cocaine Frequency, Race-White, Sex Exchange Risk Partners. Includes subjects who reported sexual activity both in-treatment and pre-treatment.
4. Definition of this variable excludes needle-sharing patners for the Sexual Partner Risk Composite regression.

cantly correlated individually with the sex partner risk composite), so that an interaction term representing this combination was included in the regression analysis. Factors associated with the sexual partner risk composite score at in-treatment were: total treatment/detoxification admissions, drug sales offenses, heavy alcohol use, the ASPD × white interaction effect and sexual partner risk composite score at pre-treatment. Factors associated with unprotected sex at in-treatment were: fewer drug sales offenses, being female, less education, fewer drug risk sex partners and unprotected sex at pre-treatment.

Validity of Self-Reports

The accuracy of drug use self-reports by persons at risk for use varies widely among different studies and drug user populations.[37,38] According to these reviews, however, patients enrolled in methadone treatment report their drug use to researchers with moderate to high degrees of accuracy. Nevertheless, confidence in the current study's results would be increased if some additional evidence for the validity of the patient self-reports could be obtained.

There are no means of directly validating self-reports of HIV risk behaviors. However, an indirect approach is feasible in this study, which involves comparing self-reports of heroin use with clinic urinalyses for the month preceding the interview. Patients who are found to report heroin use inaccurately, for whatever reason, may also be reporting HIV risk behaviors inaccurately. Up to four urinalyses were available for the month preceding the interview. The apparent discrepancies were as follows: eighteen percent of the patients reported no heroin or other opiate use, but had an opiate-positive urine ("underreporters"), and 12% of the patients reported opiate use, but had no opiate-positive urines ("overreporters").

Since there seems to be no reason for patients to report opiates when not using them, the apparent "overreporting" is probably due to some opiate use not being detected through the average of about three urinalyses per month found for this group. Underreporting is a potentially more serious problem, since it could be associated with lower reporting of in-treatment HIV behaviors and thus could lead to an overstatement of HIV risk reduction for the sample. The influence of possible underreporting was examined by repeating the paired pre- versus in-treatment comparisons for the HIV risk measures with exclusion of the apparent opiate underreporters. The results were nearly identical to the analyses with the full sample; all previously significant associations remained significant.

DISCUSSION AND CONCLUSIONS

Methadone patients who continue to use cocaine nonetheless show substantial reductions in needle-related and sexually-related HIV risk behaviors during treatment; this supports prior research.[11] Many methadone programs discharge patients for continuing cocaine use or for treatment non-compliance associated with such use.[39] This probably results in patients' return to pre-treatment levels of heroin use, injection frequency and other HIV risk behaviors. (Outcomes for methadone patients who leave treatment are very poor.[4]) A better policy from a public health perspective is to maintain cocaine users in treatment, unless their behavior is truly disruptive to the program (e.g., trading in drugs on or near the premises, threatening staff).

Of course cocaine/crack use is inconsistent with a long-term goal of recovery from drug addiction. Research must continue on behavioral and pharmacological therapies for cocaine dependence/abuse among both primary cocaine users and methadone patients. In the interim, patients' access to harm reduction methods such as needle exchange and free condoms should be increased.[12,40]

Although HIV risk behaviors declined substantially for the patients after admission, there were no apparent time in treatment effects, i.e., patient length of treatment was not associated with differences in risk behaviors at the time of the interview. This might be because changes occur fairly rapidly after entry to treatment (as early as three months later, as previously reported,[11] and/or because those least likely to change drop out early and are underrepresented in our in-treatment sample. Bux et al. (1995) also found that time in treatment was unrelated to injection frequency for a methadone sample that included both cocaine users and non-users.[29] Grella et al. (1996), who prospectively followed up a sample of new female admissions to methadone maintenance, found that women who stayed in treatment at least one year had greater reductions in sex partners and needle-sharing partners.[15]

Needle hygiene risks, which were relevant to only a small number of patients still sharing paraphernalia, did not change during treatment. This may point to the practical difficulties of effective needle cleaning in typical injection settings and, consequently, the importance of needle exchanges or other means of access to legal (including free) needles.[41]

There were different predictors of change for injection frequency and needle sharing risk. The predictors of the needle risk composite score, as might be expected, included predictors from both domains. Heroin use frequency was the strongest predictor of injection frequency because injection is the preferred route of administration for heroin in this population. Anti-social personality disorder (ASPD) also predicted injection frequency, a result consistent with two prior studies.[42,43] In contrast, another study found no association between ASPD and drug injection for an Australian methadone sample, although an association was found between injection and a global measure of psychopathology.[30]

In two previous studies, ASPD was found to be associated with needle-sharing for methadone patients,[42,43] although not by a third study[44] or the current research. One possible explanation for this discrepancy might be the difference in time frames; the first two studies asked about sharing during the past year, while the last two asked about sharing during the past six months and past month, respectively. Since rates of sharing seemed to be relatively low, it may be that differences will only emerge for longer time intervals.

The association of current bipolar disorder with continued injection during treatment apparently has not been reported previously. Bipolar disorder responds to medications and, given this finding, should receive high priority for diagnosis and treatment

The association of violent behavior with needle sharing also has not been reported previously (apparently no past studies have examined this), although several studies found various indices of criminal activity to be associated independently with needle-sharing;[15,30,45] "this may indicate greater entrenchment in a risky lifestyle." [30]

Needle sharing was not associated with having drug risk sexual partners, contradicting previous findings.[30,45,15] Overlapping definitions of these variables could lead to tautological findings. However, women were more likely to report sharing in the current study, which is consistent with a prior study.[11] This underscores the importance of expanding targeted HIV preventive interventions for female methadone patients.[46,47]

HIV seropositivity was associated with needle sharing; another study also found a trend ($p < .10$) toward an association between HIV seropositivity and needle-sharing partners (including sexual and non-sexual partners).[15] Note that in both studies, knowledge of seropositivity preceded the period in which sharing was measured. Although those who know they are seropositive might be anticipated to refrain from sharing injection equipment, there are several reasons why they might be more likely to share, such as: an inability to break a habit which contributed to their HIV infection in the first place, a belief that avoiding HIV infection has become irrelevant, or sharing only with others who are HIV positive. Clearly this finding, in conjunction with a previous study,[48] raises questions about the effectiveness of HIV testing and post-test counseling in reducing HIV transmission among injecting drug users.

The predictors of sexual partner risk and unprotected sex tended to be different. Several variables were associated with sex partner risk. Total treatment/detoxification admissions probably indicate longer and more extensive drug use involvement. Heavy alcohol use might have a disinhibiting effect for sex with many partners or high risk partners; another study reports a similar association.[15] Alcohol abuse could be addressed in methadone programs by 12-step facilitation efforts.

White subjects with ASPD might be a unique group immersed in a particularly risky lifestyle. ASPD diagnosis may have a different meaning for white vs. minority group drug users. The latter may be more susceptible to meeting adolescent and adult ASPD criteria (as behaviorally defined on the SCID) because of the often greater disorganization and police surveillance of their communities. Consequently white as compared with minority drug users diagnosed with ASPD may have a relatively more severe disorder; one manifestation of this greater severity could be more sexual activity with high risk partners. Another study found that white female methadone patients reported more sexual partners than minority female patients, although a possible link with ASPD could not be explored[15]. (However, white ASPD subjects in the current study were not more likely to report unprotected sex.)

The various associations between ASPD and HIV risk behaviors in the current study suggest that greater efforts should be made to diagnose ASPD and intensify services to such patients. There is unfortunately no tested therapeutic model available; clinical research is needed in this area.

Females and patients with less education were more likely to engage in unprotected sex, possibly because females are disadvantaged in negotiating condom use and because of socioeconomically-based attitudes against such use. The inverse association of unprotected sex with drug risk sex partners may be attributable to a desire for protection against HIV; another study reported a similar finding.[15] Finally, those involved in drug selling are more likely to have protected sex; possibly they are considered by others to be riskier sexual partners and thus are asked to use condoms. This interpretation would be consistent with the previous finding that having drug risk sex partners is associated with condom use.

The apparent opiate use underreporting requires some comment, since all these patients were admitted cocaine/crack users. Although the interview did inquire about "pill use," complete data might not have been obtained on all codeine-containing pills and compounds that patients may have taken with or without prescription, e.g., the interview did not explicitly ask about cough syrup with codeine. It is also possible that patients ingesting some opiate-containing pills or cough syrup may not have considered themselves "using" or "taking" these substances. In any event, the exclusion of apparent opiate underreporters from the pre- vs. in-treatment analysis of changes in HIV risk behaviors did not alter the results. Another study performed a similar analysis of drug use reporting validity for methadone patients with findings similar to those presented here.[12]

Study Limitations

Because reports of pre-treatment behaviors were retrospective–an average of two years ago–the accuracy of subjects' recall can be questioned. However, the reports were linked to a distinct salient event, admission to methadone treatment, which should improve accuracy of recall. To place this in context, in many studies, including the current one, subjects are asked routinely to recall events and behaviors even further removed in time, e.g., information needed for lifetime DSM diagnoses.

The generalizability of findings may be limited, since subjects were sampled from only one methadone program.

No measures of ancillary services or intensity of services after admission to methadone treatment were available that might have affected the prevalence of HIV risk behaviors during treatment.

The analyses presented are correlational and, although causal interpretations were sometimes made, these must be considered tentative.

REFERENCES

1. Simpson DD, Sells SB. Effectiveness of treatment for drug abuse: An overview of the DARP research program. Adv Alcohol Subst Abuse 1982; 2:7-29.

2. Anglin MD, McGlothlin WH. Outcome of narcotic addict treatment in California. In: Tims F and Ludford J, eds. Drug abuse treatment evaluation: Strategies, progress and prospects. NIDA Res Monogr. 51. Rockville, MD: National Insitute on Drug Abuse, 1984.

3. Hubbard RL, Marsden ME, Rachal JV, Harwood HJ, Cavanaugh ER, Ginzburg HM. Drug abuse treatment: A national study of effectiveness. Chapel Hill, NC: University of North Carolina Press, 1989.

4. Ball JC, Ross A. The effectiveness of methadone maintenance treatment. New York: Springer-Varlag 1991.

5. Abdul-Quader AS, Friedman SR, Des Jarlais D, Marmor MM, Maslansky R, Bartelme S. Methadone maintenance and behavior by intravenous drug users that can transmit HIV. Contemporary Drug Problems 1987; 14:425-434.

6. Ball JC, Lange RW, Myers PC, Friedman SR. Reducing the risk of AIDS through methadone maintenance treatment. J Health Social Beh. 1988; 29: 214-226.

7. Hubbard RL, Marsden ME, Cavanaugh E, Rachal JV, Ginzburg HM. Role of drug abuse treatment in limiting the spread of AIDS. Rev of Infect Dis. 1988; 10: 377-384.

8. Gottheil E, Sterling RC, Weinstein SP. Diminished illicit drug use as a consequence of long-term methadone maintenance. J Addict Dis. 1993; 12:45-57.

9. Longshore D, Hsieh SC, Danila B, Anglin MD. Methadone maintenance and needle/syringe sharing. Int J Addict. 1993; 28:983-996.

10. Capelhorn JR, Ross MW. Methadone maintenance and the likelihood of risky needle-sharing. Int J Addict. 1995; 30:685-698.

11. Camacho LM, Bartholomew NG, Joe GW, Cloud MA, Simpson DD. Gender, cocaine and during-treatment HIV risk reduction among injection opioid users in methadone maintenance. Drug Alcohol Depend. 1996; 41:1-7.

12. Hartel DM, Schoenbaum EE, Selwyn PA, Friedland GH, Klein RS, Drucker E. Patterns of heroin, cocaine and speedball injection among Bronx (USA) methadone maintenance patients: 1978-1988. Addiction Research 1996; 3 (4): 323-340.

13. Magura S, Shapiro J, Siddiqi Q, Lipton DS. Variables influencing condom use among IV drug users. Am J Public Health 1990; 80 (1): 82-84.

14. Watkins KE, Metzger D, Woody G, McLellan AT. High-risk sexual behaviors of intravenous drug users in- and out-of-treatment; implications for the spread of HIV infection. Am J Drug Alcohol Abuse, 1992; 18:389-398

15. Grella CE, Anglin MD, Annon JJ. HIV risk behaviors among women in methadone maintenance treatment. Subst Use & Misuse 1996; 31 (3): 277-301.

16. Marmor M, Des Jarlais DC, Cohen H, Friedman SR, Beatrice ST, Dubin N, El-Sadr W, Mildvan D, Yancovitz S, Mathur U, Holzman R. Risk factors for infection with human immunodeficiency virus among intravenous drug abusers in New York City. AIDS 1987; 1:39-44.

17. Barthwell A, Senay E, Marks R, White R. Patients successfully maintained with methadone escaped human immunodeficiency virus infection. Arch Gen Psychiatry 1989; 46:957-958.

18. Chaisson RE, Bacchetti P, Osmong E, Brodie B, Sande M and Moss A. Cocaine use and HIV infection in intravenous drug users in San Francisco. J Am Med Assoc. 1989; 261:561-565.

19. West AP. Drug abuse treatment as a strategy to prevent human immunodeficiency virus infection among intravenous drug abusers. Arch Intern Med. 1991; 151: 1493-1496.

20. Cooper JR. Methadone treatment and acquired immunodeficiency syndrome. J Am Med Assoc. 1989; 262:1664-1668.

21. Novick DM, Joseph H, Croxson TS, et al. Absence of antibody to human immunodeficiency virus in long-term, socially rehabilitated methadone maintenance patients. Arch Intern Med. 1990; 150:97-99.

22. Kosten TR, Rounsaville BJ. Cocaine abuse among opioid addicts. Am J Drug Alcohol Abuse 1986; 12:1-16.

23. Strain EC, Stitzer ML, Liebson IA, Bigelow GE. Outcome after methadone treatment: Influence of prior treatment factors and current treatment status. Drug Alcohol Depend. 1994; 35: 223-230.

24. Magura S, Siddiqi Q, Freeman RC, Lipton DS. Changes in cocaine use after entry to methadone treatment. J Addict Dis. 1991; 4:31-25.

25. Magura S, Siddiqi Q, Freeman RC, Lipton DS. Cocaine use and help-seeking among methadone patients. J Drug Issues 1991; 21:629-645.

26. Torrens M, San L, Peri JM, Olle JM. Cocaine abuse among heroin addicts in Spain. Drug Alcohol Depend. 1991; 27:29-32.

27. Iguchi MY, Platt JJ, French J, Baxter RC, Kushner H, Lidz VM, Bux DA, Rosen M, Musikoff H. Correlates of HIV seropositivity among injection drug users not in treatment. J Drug Issues 1992; 22 (4):849-866.

28. Nemoto T. Patterns of cocaine use and HIV infection among injection drug users in a methadone clinic. J Subst Abuse 1994; 6 (2):169-178.

29. Bux DA, Lamb RJ, Iguchi MY. Cocaine use and HIV risk behavior in methadone maintenance patients. Drug Alcohol Depend. 1995; 37:29-35.

30. Darke S, Baker A, Dixon J, Wodak A, Heather N. Drug use and HIV risk-taking behaviour among clients in methadone maintenance treatment. Drug Alcohol Depend. 1992; 29:263-268.

31. Magura S, Rosenblum A, Lovejoy M, Foote J, Handelsman L, Stimmel B. Neurobehavioral treatment for cocaine-using methadone patients: preliminary report. J Addict Dis. 1994; 13:143-160.

32. Spitzer RL, Williams JBW, Gibbon M, First MB. Structured Clinical Interview for DSM-III-R-Patient Edition (With Psychotic Screen). Washington, DC, American Psychiatric Press, 1990.

33. Derogatis LR. The Brief Symptom Inventory. Baltimore: Clinical Psychometric Research, 1975.

34. Norusis MJ. SPSS Base System Users Guide. Chicago, SPSS, Inc. 1990.

35. Magura S, Kang SY, Rosenblum A, Handelsman L, Foote J. Gender differences in psychiatric comorbidity among cocaine-using opiate addicts. J Addict Dis., 1998; 17(3):49-61.

36. Derogatis LR, Spencer PM. Brief Symptom Inventory. Administration & Procedures: BSI Manual-I. Baltimore: Clinical Psychometric Research Inc., 1982.

37. Magura S, Kang SY. Validity of self-reported drug use in high risk populations: A meta-analytical review. Subst Use and Misuse 1996; 31 (9):1131-1153.

38. Magura S, Goldsmith DC, Castriel C et al. The validity of methadone clients' self-reported drug use. Int J Addict. 1987; 22 (8): 727-749.

39. Kolar AF, Brown BS, Weddington WW, Ball JC. A treatment crisis: cocaine use by clients in methadone maintenance programs. J Subst Abuse Treat. 1990; 7: 101-107.

40. Magura S, Grossman J, Lipton DS et al. Determinants of needle-sharing among intravenous drug users. Am J Public Health 1989; 79 (4):459-462.

41. McCusker J, Stoddard AM, Koblin B, Sullivan J, Lewis BF, Seteti M. Time trends in high-risk injection practices in a multi-site study in Massachusetts: Effects of enrollment site and residence. AIDS Educ Prev. 1992; 4 (2):108-119.

42. Gill K, Nolimal D, Crowley T. Antisocial personality disorder: HIV risk behavior and retention in methadone maintenane therapy. Drug Alcohol Depend 1992; 30:247-252.

43. Brooner RK, Greenfield LG, Schmidt CW, Bigelow GE. Antisocial personality disorder and HIV infection in intravenous drug abusers. Am J Psychiatry 1993; 1: 53-58.

44. Abbott PJ, Weller SB, Walker SR. Psychiatric disorders of opioid addicts entering treatment: Preliminary data. J Addict Dis. 1994; 13 (3):1-11.

45. Donoghoe MC, Dolan KA, Stimson GV. Life-style factors and social circumstances of syringe sharing in injecting drug users. Br J Addict. 1992; 87:993-1003.

46. Bartholomew N, Rowan-Szal GA, Chatham LR, Simpson DD. Effectiveness of a specialized intervention for women in a methadone program. J Psychoactive Drugs 1994; 29:249-255.

47. El-Bassel N, Schilling RF. 15-month follow-up of women methadone patients taught skills to reduce heterosexual HIV transmission. Public Health Rep. 1992; 107: 500-504.

48. Calsyn DA, Saxon G, Freeman G, Whitaker. Ineffectiveness of AIDS education and HIV antibody testing in reducing high risk behaviors among injection drug users. Am J Public Health 1992; 82:573-575.

HIV/AIDS and Drug Abuse: Epidemiology and Prevention

Harry W. Haverkos, MD

SUMMARY. In the United States, the AIDS epidemic is a dynamic process with increasing rates of AIDS reported among women, minority populations, heterosexual men, and users of drugs by routes other than injection. The 1993 CDC AIDS definition change has created some difficulties in interpreting trends in the United States. Drug use continues to represent a significant problem among HIV-infected persons. Several strategies have been advanced to decrease transmission of HIV among drug users, their sexual partners and children. However, more effective and comprehensive prevention and treatment strategies are needed. *[Article copies available for a fee from The Haworth Document Delivery Service: 1-800-342-9678. E-mail address: getinfo@haworthpressinc.com]*

EPIDEMIOLOGY: WHERE IS THE EPIDEMIC GOING?

During the 1970s and early 1980s, the HIV/AIDS epidemic spread rapidly among the homosexual male population in the United States and Europe.[1,2] This early phase of the pandemic was followed closely by a second wave of

Harry W. Haverkos, at the time of this study, was affiliated with the Intramural Research Program, National Institute on Drug Abuse, National Institutes of Health, Rockville, MD. Currently he is Medical Officer, HFD-530, Food and Drug Administration, 5600 Fishers Lane, Rockville, MD 20857.

The author would like to thank Drs. Steve Gust, Richard Needle, Wallace Pickworth, and Annie Umbricht for reviewing drafts of the paper and offering comments.

[Haworth co-indexing entry note]: "HIV/AIDS and Drug Abuse: Epidemiology and Prevention." Haverkos, Harry W. Co-published simultaneously in *Journal of Addictive Diseases* (The Haworth Medical Press, an imprint of The Haworth Press, Inc.) Vol. 17, No. 4, 1998, pp. 91-103; and: *Effects of Substance Abuse Treatment on AIDS Risk Behaviors* (ed: Edward Gottheil, and Barry Stimmel) The Haworth Medical Press, an imprint of The Haworth Press, Inc., 1998, pp. 91-103. Single or multiple copies of this article are available for a fee from The Haworth Document Delivery Service [1-800-342-9678, 9:00 a.m. - 5:00 p.m. (EST). E-mail address: getinfo@haworthpressinc.com].

HIV/AIDS among injecting drug users.[3] Shortly thereafter, there was widespread recognition that AIDS was occurring among heterosexuals residing in developing countries of Africa and the Caribbean. The "third wave" of HIV infection among heterosexuals was appreciated more recently in large metropolitan areas of the United States and Europe.[4,5]

All three waves of the pandemic have been highly associated with drug abuse. Although rates of HIV seroincidence and AIDS deaths are declining among white gay men in large urban areas of the USA, increases are seen among gay men of color in urban areas and among gay men in smaller cities and rural areas. Several epidemiologic studies have shown increased HIV infection risk among gay men who use drugs, such as alcohol, amphetamines, cocaine, and nitrite inhalants.[6-9] HIV infection and AIDS among injecting drug users have been reported on every continent, especially in the eastern United States, Puerto Rico, and parts of Europe, especially Italy, Spain, and Switzerland. A survey of public health officials in 96 of the largest metropolitan areas in the US revealed that injection drug users accounted for roughly half of all new HIV infections.[10] Worldwide, the most explosive rates of new HIV infections have been reported among injection drug users in the "Golden Triangle" and surrounding areas of Asia known for their production of heroin.[11,12] HIV infection rates among heterosexuals who do not inject, but who use drugs, such as amphetamines and cocaine, by other routes of administration, are also increasing in several parts of the US.[13-15]

Between June 1981 and December 31, 1996, 581,429 patients with AIDS in the USA and territories have been reported to the Centers for Disease Control and Prevention (CDC), Atlanta. Effective January 1, 1993, the CDC changed the definition of AIDS, which has created difficulties monitoring recent trends in the epidemic. The number of AIDS cases reported in 1994 (80,691), 1995 (74,180) and 1996 (69,151) declined from the number reported in 1993 (106,618), the year the expanded definition was employed. The 1993 numbers of AIDS cases was significantly higher than the number reported in 1992 (45,572). Because the trends for recent years may be distorted, additional methods are needed to adjust for the case definition change.[16]

One method to assess trends is to compare rates of AIDS among various populations.[17] From such comparisons the HIV epidemic appears to be a dynamic process. The change in characteristics of persons with AIDS can be documented by comparing the rates in the early years of the epidemic with those reported in more recent years. (Note: Tables 1 and 2 compare years 1981-1988 with data from 1996, but similar results can be documented comparing any combinations of early years with more recent year data). The fastest growing groups of patients are women, African-Americans, Hispanics, and heterosexuals who do not inject drugs.[16]

TABLE 1. Changes in Characteristics of Persons Reported with AIDS: Comparison of 1981-1988 with 1996.

	1981-1988		1996		Change in Proportion of Cases Over Time*
	N	%	N	%	%
Adults/Adolescents					
Sex					
Male	74,435	91.4	54,653	79.8	− 12.7
Female	6,983	8.6	13,820	20.2	+134.9
Race/Ethnicity					
White	47,307	58.1	26,229	38.3	− 34.1
African-American	21,222	26.1	28,346	41.4	+58.6
Hispanic	12,133	14.9	12,966	18.9	+26.8
Other*	569	0.7	768	1.1	+57.1
Exposure Category					
MSM	50,325	61.8	27,316	39.5	− 36.1
IDU					
Male	15,529	19.1	12,333	17.8	− 6.8
Female	3,622	4.4	4,694	6.8	+54.5
MSM/IDU	5,874	7.2	2,967	4.3	− 40.3
Heterosexual contact					
Male	1,499	1.8	3,299	4.8	+166.7
Female	2,059	2.5	5,522	8.0	+220.0
Hemophiliac	773	0.9	318	0.5	− 44.4
Transfusion recipient	2,044	2.5	551	0.8	− 68.0
No Risk Reported	2,693	3.3	11,473	16.8	N/A**
Pediatric (< 13 years)	1,346	1.6	678	0.9	− 43.8

[Modification of Table in Reference 17]
*Change in Proportion over Time determined by subtracting 1996% from 1981-88% divided by 1981-88%. For example, Change for Female IDUs is 1996% (6.8) minus 1981-88% (4.4) divided by 1981-88% (4.4) equals plus 54.5%.
**See text

(Note: The group "No Risk Reported" shows marked increases over time, but comparisons for this group are fraught with difficulties of interpretation. For example, investigators have had more time to evaluate and categorize patients from earlier time periods than those reported in recent years. Unfortunately, State health departments and the CDC collect little or no data regarding nonprescription or illicit drug use by routes other than injection. Many investigators believe that heterosexual transmission of HIV associated with alcohol, cocaine, and other drugs accounts for a significant number of

TABLE 2. Changes in Distribution of Persons with AIDS from the 20 US Metropolitan Areas Reporting the Largest Numbers of Patients: Comparison of 1981-1988 with 1996.

	1981-1988		1996		Change in Proportion of Cases Over Time
	N	%	N	%	%
Atlanta	1,430	1.7	1,642	2.4	+41.2
Baltimore	748	0.9	1,525	2.2	+144.4
Boston	1,391	1.7	1,102	1.6	−5.9
Chicago	2,022	2.4	1,841	2.6	+8.3
Dallas	1,459	1.8	892	1.3	−27.8
Detroit	652	0.8	706	1.0	+25.0
Ft. Lauderdale	1,023	1.2	1,203	1.7	+41.7
Houston	2,544	3.1	1,719	2.5	−19.4
Los Angeles	6,012	7.3	3,716	5.4	−26.0
Miami	2,092	2.5	2,063	3.0	+20.0
New York	17,684	21.4	10,385	15.0	−29.9
Newark	2,414	2.9	1,434	2.1	−27.6
Oakland	1,011	1.2	629	0.9	−25.0
Philadelphia	1,674	2.0	1,679	2.4	+20.0
San Diego	1,131	1.4	984	1.4	No Change
San Juan	977	1.2	1,395	2.0	+66.7
San Francisco	5,626	6.8	1,572	2.3	−66.2
Tampa-St. Petersburg	746	0.9	793	1.1	+22.2
Washington	2,404	2.9	2,160	3.1	+8.3
West Palm Beach	733	0.8	848	1.2	+50.0
Top 20 Metro Areas	53,773	65.0	38,288	55.4	−14.8
Other Metros (>50K)	17,897	21.6	25,692	37.2	+72.2
Non-Metro	11,094	13.4	5,171	7.5	−44.0
Total	82,764	100.0	69,151	100.0	N/A

patients listed in the "No Risk Reported" category, but are unable to prove that contention using national data.)

In fact, the number of heterosexual contact AIDS patients is increasing in all ages, ethnic groups, and geographic regions. There is also a shift occurring among risk factors of sex partners of heterosexual AIDS patients. Initially sexual contact with an HIV-infected drug user was the most common mode of acquisition among heterosexuals with AIDS. Now the fastest growing subset of heterosexual patients is one linked to HIV-infected partners whose risk is not specified, suggesting that secondary and tertiary HIV transmission is occurring beyond the original "high-risk" groups.[16]

Although AIDS was first reported in Los Angeles, New York City, and San Francisco, the disease has rapidly spread throughout the USA. Table 2 lists changes in the distribution of persons with AIDS in the 20 US metropolitan areas reporting the largest numbers of patients. Although those 20 metropolitan areas still report over half the cases of AIDS in the US, the fastest growing rates are occurring in many smaller cities throughout the country.[16]

In summary, HIV disease burden in the USA remains greatest among men who have sex with men and injecting drug abusers, but is growing most rapidly among minorities, women, and heterosexuals. Sexual transmission of HIV among homosexual men and heterosexual women and men associated with non-injection illicit drug use is a major concern.

PREVENTION: WHAT CAN WE DO ABOUT IT?

Contrary to popular belief, drug users can and will change behaviors to decrease their risk of HIV infection. In fact, several prevention strategies have been studied by NIDA grantees and have shown significant behavior change and/or decreased HIV transmission rates among participants. However, it is also clear, at this time, that no single intervention will solve the complex, HIV/AIDS problem among injecting, non-injecting drug users, their sexual contacts and children–there is no "magic bullet."

DRUG ABUSE TREATMENT AND MEDICATIONS DEVELOPMENT

Methadone maintenance therapy has consistently lowered rates of risky needle-sharing behaviors and HIV transmission among opiate dependent populations.[18-22] In 1985 New York investigators reported that drug users with chronic liver disease in methadone programs had one-half the HIV prevalence as those with chronic liver disease who were currently not in drug abuse treatment. In fact, those in treatment for at least five years and reporting no needle use during that time had an HIV rate one-tenth that of those not in treatment.[18] In Philadelphia, researchers compared HIV incidence and risk behaviors of drug abusers in methadone maintenance with those out-of-treatment in a prospective study. They found lower rates of HIV seroincidence, needle-sharing, injection frequency, shooting gallery use, and visits to crack houses among the methadone-maintained IDUs.[19]

Despite those results, there has been little support for expanding drug abuse treatment programs and facilities for opiate addicts in the USA. It is estimated that only about fifteen percent of injecting opiate users are currently in drug abuse treatment.[20] In addition, abusers other substances, such as cocaine and amphetamines, are at risk for HIV infection and treatment options are limited for them.[22,23]

The Medications Development Division (MDD) of the National Institute on Drug Abuse (NIDA) was established in 1991 to support research to rapidly study medications for treatment of opiate and cocaine dependency. Enhancing the research infrastructure during the past six years has led to the Food and Drug Administration approval of LAAM, another opiate agonist option available for heroin abusers.[24,25] Additionally this infrastructure has established a discovery system for identification of potential medications for cocaine treatment and a system to rapidly test such agents in clinical trials.

Although there is no pharmacotherapy with demonstrated efficacy in the treatment of cocaine addiction, there are behavioral therapies showing promise.[26,27] One approach is called community reinforcement, which is contingency contracting between counselor and patient and also between significant other and patient with incentives provided for documentation of drug-free urinalyses. In a randomized study, community reinforcement led to greater cocaine abstinence and longer retention rates than self-help therapy.[26]

COMMUNITY-BASED OUTREACH RISK REDUCTION PROJECTS

It is estimated that the vast majority (50-85%) of injecting drug users are not in drug abuse treatment programs at any point in time. To limit the spread of HIV infection among injecting drug users, communities have relied on outreach to IDUs to create opportunities to counsel addicts about HIV infection and AIDS. Outreach interventions consist of risk-reduction information and referral to drug treatment and other services, condom and bleach distribution, HIV antibody testing, pre- and posttest counseling, and demonstration and rehearsal of risk reduction skills. Generally, IDUs who receive those interventions reduce their needle-related risk behaviors to some degree during followup. Sexual behavior change has been more difficult to document in those studies.[28-30]

BLEACH DISINFECTION OF NEEDLES/SYRINGES

The history of bleach disinfection of needles as an outreach intervention demonstrates the important interaction of basic science and behavioral research to evaluate strategies for HIV prevention. In initial laboratory studies, bleach was found to inactivate HIV in laboratory samples. Bleach became a point of contact with out-of-treatment IDUs to provide AIDS education and recruit for drug abuse treatment.[31]

Further basic science and epidemiologic research led to a realization that bleach was limited in its antiretroviral activity under field conditions. Ongoing research will define conditions necessary to completely inactivate HIV in needles/syringes. These observations about bleach led to studies to define the role of other injection paraphernalia in HIV transmission ("indirect sharing"), i.e., cookers, cottons, and rinse water. It also spurred research for other needle hygiene interventions and "risk reduction" approaches, such as, needle/syringe exchange and revision of drug paraphernalia laws.[31]

NEEDLE/SYRINGE EXCHANGE

In an effort to reach injecting drug users who continue to place themselves and others at risk, a number of communities across the United States and abroad have initiated needle/syringe exchange programs in the hope that increased availability of sterile needles/syringes will reduce needle sharing. Although drug abuse treatment remains the primary means of reducing HIV risk among drug abusers, it has now been shown that much can be accomplished with addicts not yet able or willing to enter treatment, and needle/syringe exchange may be a safe and useful component of a comprehensive HIV prevention program.[32-34] Negative consequences of increased needle/syringe availability must be studied.

FUTURE RESEARCH

What are the most important directions to pursue in drug abuse research to have the greatest impact on HIV transmission? In my opinion, there are three areas or goals that would have great impact on HIV transmission among drug users.

The cocaine epidemic of the 1980s put both injectors and non-injectors of drugs at greater risk for HIV infection. Finding an effective pharmacologic therapy for cocaine and other stimulants would be most helpful.

Although NIDA grantees have shown some success altering needle-sharing behaviors and decreasing HIV transmission through a number of strategies, negligible effects have been seen altering sexual behaviors of drug users. Heterosexual transmission of HIV is the fastest growing exposure category throughout the world, including the United States and Europe. Finding an effective behavioral intervention to decrease sexual transmission of HIV among sexually active drug users, both for homosexual and heterosexual individuals, would go far in stemming HIV transmission. It will also be important to develop and promote comprehensive prevention programs to alter both needle-sharing, drug-using, and sexual behaviors among both HIV-infected and non-infected individuals.

Finally, there are three recently published Federal documents that focus on different aspects of the problem(s). The intent of the documents differ. The Office of National Drug Control Policy in *The National Drug Control Strategy* (Table 3) focuses on prevention of drug use, emphasizing different strategies from demand reduction targeted to special population, i.e., adolescents, to interdiction of supplies. The NIH Consensus Development Conference Statement on *Intervention to Prevent HIV Risk Behaviors* (Table 4) reviewed evidence on the effectiveness of interdictions for prevention and made recommendations to prevent further spread of HIV among several populations, including drug abusers. The U.S. Public Health Service HIV Prevention Bulletin (Table 5) made recommendations for drug using populations at highest risk for HIV, those who continue to inject drugs of abuse. Its goals

TABLE 3. Strategic Goals and Selected Objectives of the 1997 National Drug Control Strategy, by the White House and Office of National Drug Control Policy, February 1997.

Goal 1: Educate and enable America's youth to reject illegal drugs as well as alcohol and tobacco. (Ten objectives)

Goal 2: Increase the safety of America's citizens by substantially reducing drug-related crime and violence. (Six objectives)

Goal 3: Reduce health and social costs to the public of illegal drug use.
    Objective 1: Support and promote effective, efficient, and accessible drug treatment, ensuring the development of a system that is responsive to emerging trends in drug abuse.
    Objective 2: Reduce drug-related health problems, with an emphasis on infectious diseases.
    Objective 3: Promote national adoption of drug-free workplace programs that emphasize drug testing as a key component of a comprehensive program that includes education, prevention, and intervention.
    Objective 4: Support and promote the education, training, and credentialing of professionals who work with substance abusers.
    Objective 5: Support research into the development of medications and treatment protocols to prevent or reduce drug dependence and abuse.
    Objective 6: Support and highlight research and technology, including the acquisition and analysis of scientific data, to reduce the health and social costs of illegal drug use.

Goal 4: Shield America's air, land, and sea frontiers from the drug threat. (Four objectives)

Goal 5: Break foreign and domestic drug sources of supply. (Six objectives)
- - - - - -
[See Reference 35]

TABLE 4. Conclusions and Recommendations, National Institutes of Health Consensus Development Conference Statement, Interventions to Prevent HIV Risk Behaviors, February 11-13, 1997.

1. Preventive interventions are effective for reducing behavioral risk for HIV/AIDS and must be widely disseminated. Their application in practice settings may require careful training of personnel, close monitoring of the fidelity of procedures, and ongoing monitoring of effectiveness. Results of this evaluation must be reported; and where effectiveness in field settings is reduced, program modifications must be undertaken immediately.

Three approaches are particularly effective for risk in drug abuse behavior: needle exchange programs, drug abuse treatment, and outreach programs for drug abusers not enrolled in treatment. Several programs were deemed to be effective for risky sexual behavior. These programs include (1) information about HIV/AIDS and (2) building skills to use condoms and to negotiate the interpersonal challenges of safe sex. Effective safe sex programs have been developed for men who have sex with men, for women, and for adolescents.

2. The epidemic in the United States is shifting to young people, particularly those who are gay and who are members of ethnic minority groups. New research must focus on these emerging groups. Interventions must be developed and perfected, and special attention must be given to long-term maintenance of effects. In addition, AIDS is steadily increasing in women, and transmission of HIV to their children remains a major public health problem. Interventions focused on their special needs are essential.

3. Regional tracking of changes in behavioral risk is necessary to identify settings, subpopulations, and geographical regions with special risk for seroconversion to HIV-positive status as the epidemic continues to change. This effort, if properly coordinated with National tracking strategies, could play a critical part in a U.S. strategy to contain the spread of HIV.

4. Programs must be developed to help individuals already infected with HIV to avoid risky sexual and substance abuse behavior. This National priority will become more pressing as new biological treatments prolong life. Thus, prevention programs for HIV-positive people must have outcomes that can be maintained over long periods of time, in order to slow the spread of infection.

5. Legislative restriction on needle exchange programs must be lifted. Such legislation constitutes a major barrier to realizing the potential of a powerful approach and exposes millions of people to unnecessary risk.

6. Legislative barriers that discourage effective programs aimed at youth must be eliminated. Although sexual abstinence is a desirable objective, programs must include instruction in safe sex behavior, including condom use. The effectiveness of these programs is supported by strong scientific evidence. However, they are discouraged by welfare reform provisions, which support only programs using abstinence as the only goal.

7. The erosion of funding for drug and alcohol abuse treatment programs must be halted. Research data are clear that the programs reduce risky drug and alcohol abuse behavior and often eliminate drug abuse itself. Drug and alcohol abuse treatment is a central bulwark in the Nation's defense against HIV/AIDS.

8. The catastrophic breach between HIV/AIDS prevention science and legislative process must be healed. Citizens, legislators, political leaders, service providers, and scientists must unite so that scientific data may properly inform legislative process. The study of policy development, the impact of policy, and policy change must be supported by Federal agencies.

- - - - - -

[See Reference 36]

TABLE 5. Provisional Recommendations to Drug Users Who Continue to Inject. HIV Prevention Bulletin, by the Centers for Disease Control and Prevention, Health Resources & Services Administration, National Institute on Drug Abuse, and Substance Abuse and Mental Health Services Administration, May 9, 1997.

Health care workers involved in programs that serve drug users should communicate the following recommendations to drug users who continue to inject. Adhering to these drug preparation and injection procedures will reduce the public health and individual health risks associated with drug injection for both drug users and other persons in their communities.
Persons who inject drugs should be regularly counseled to:

I. Stop using and injecting drugs.

II. Enter and complete substance abuse treatment, including relapse prevention.

III. Take the following steps to reduce personal and public health risks, if they continue to inject drugs:

Never reuse or "share" syringes, water, or drug preparation equipment.

Use only syringes obtained from a reliable source (e.g., pharmacies).

Use a new, sterile syringe to prepare and inject drugs.

If possible, use sterile water to prepare drugs; otherwise use clean water from a reliable source (such as fresh tap water).

Use a new or disinfected "cooker" and a new "cotton" to prepare drugs.

Clean the injection site prior to injection with a new alcohol swab.

Safely dispose of syringes after one use.

The availability of new, sterile syringes varies, depending on state and local regulations regarding the sale and possession of syringes and on other factors, such as the existence of syringe exchange programs sponsored by local HIV prevention organizations. If new, sterile syringes and other drug preparation and injection equipment are not available, then previously used equipment should be boiled or disinfected with bleach using the methods recommended in the April 1993 CDC, CSAT, NIDA Prevention Bulletin (available at no cost from the CDC National AIDS Clearinghouse [1–800–458–5231]).
In addition, drug users should be provided information on how to prevent HIV transmission through sexual contact and, for women, information on reducing the risk of mother-to-infant HIV transmission.

- - - -

Reference 37

range from risk elimination, i.e., stop using drugs, to risk reduction. It does not focus on non-injection drug.

There is a need for a comprehensive statement that includes elements from each of those reports that can guide persons through prevention of initiation into drug use and through elimination of ongoing use and minimizing medical and psychological adverse consequences of drug use, abuse and dependence. There is also an urgent need for effective strategies and guidelines to prevent sexual transmission of HIV associated with drug use.

REFERENCES

1. Centers for Disease Control, Task Force on Kaposi's sarcoma and opportunistic infections. Epidemiologic aspects of the current outbreak of Kaposi's sarcoma and opportunistic infections. N Engl J Med. 1982;306:248-252.

2. Auerbach DM, Darrow WW, Jaffe HW, Curran JW. Clusters of cases of the acquired immune deficiency syndrome: Patients linked by sexual contact. Am J Med. 1984;76:487-492.

3. Masur H, Michelis MA, Greene JP, et al. An outbreak of community-acquired *Pneumocystis carinii* pneumonia: Initial manifestation of cellular dysfunction. N Engl J Med. 1981;305:1431-1438.

4. De Vincenzi I, for the European Study Group on Heterosexual Transmission of HIV. A longitudinal study of human immunodeficiency virus transmission by heterosexual partners. N Engl J Med. 1994;331:341-346.

5. Haverkos HW, Quinn TC. The Third Wave: HIV infection among heterosexuals in the United States and Europe. Int J STDs & AIDS. 1995;6:227-232.

6. Stahl R, McKusick L, Wiley J, Coates TJ, Ostrow DG. Alcohol and drug use during sexual activity and compliance with safe sex guidelines for AIDS. Health Educ Q. 1986;13:359-371.

7. Harris NV, Thiede H, McGough JP, Gordon D. Risk factors for HIV prevention among injection drug users: Results of blinded surveys in drug treatment centers, King County, Washington 1988-1991. J Acquir Imuune Def Syndr. 1993;6:1275-1282.

8. Frosch D, Shoptaw S, Huber A, Rawson RA, Ling W. Sexual HIV risk among gay and bisexual male methamphetamine abusers. J Substance Abuse Treatment. 1996;4:1-4.

9. DiFranceisco W, Ostrow DG, Chmiel JS. Sexual adventurism, high risk behavior, and human immunodeficiency virus-1 seroconversion among the Chicago MACS-CCS Cohort, 1984 to 1992: A case-control study. Sex Transm Dis. 1996;23:453-460.

10. Holmberg SC. The estimated prevalence and incidence of HIV in 96 large US Metropolitan areas. Am J Public Health. 1996;86:642-654.

11. Des Jarlais DC. The first and second decades of AIDS among injecting drug users. Br J Addict. 1992;87:347-353.

12. Des Jarlais DC, Friedman SR, Choopanya K, Vanichseni S, Ward TP. International epidemiology of HIV and AIDS among injecting drug users. AIDS. 1992;6:1053-1068.

13a. Diaz T, Chu SY, Byers Jr. RH, et al. The types of drugs used by HIV-infected injection drug users in a multistate surveillance project: Implications for intervention. Am J Public Health. 1994;84:1971-1975.

13. Edlin BR, Irwin KL, Faruque S, et al. Intersecting epidemics: Crack cocaine and HIV infection among inner-city young adults. N Engl J Med. 1994;331:1422-1427.

14. Ratner MS (ed.). Crack Pipe as Pimp: An Ethnographic Investigation of Sex-for-Crack Exchanges. New York, Lexington Books, 1993.

15. Beebe DK, Walley E. Smokable methamphetamine ('Ice'): An old drug in a different form. Am Fam Physician. 1995;51:449-453.

16. Centers for Disease Control and Prevention. HIV/AIDS Surveillance Report, Year-end editions, 1992-1996.

17. Gourevitch MN. The epidemiology of HIV and AIDS: Current trends. Med Clinics of N America. 1996;80:1223-1238.

18. Novick DM, Kreek MJ, Des Jarlais DC, Spira TJ, Khuri ET, Ragunath J, Kalyanaraman VS, Gelb AM, Miescher A. Abstract of clinical research: Therapeutic and historical aspects. NIDA Res Monogr. 1986;67:318-320.

19. Metzger DS, Woody GE, McLellan AT, et al. Human immunodeficiency virus seroconversion among in- and out-of-treatment intravenous drug users: An 18-month prospective follow-up. J Acquir Immune Defic Syndr. 1993;6:1049-1056.

20. Ball JC, Ross A. The Effectiveness of Methadone Maintenance Treatment. New York, Springer Verlag, 1991.

21. Serpellone G, Carriere MP, Rezza G, et al. Methadone treatment as a determinant of HIV risk reduction among injecting drug users: A nested case-controlled study. AIDS Care. 1994;6:215-220.

22. Meandzija B, O'Connor PG, Fitzgerald B, Rounsaville BJ, Kosten TR. HIV infection and cocaine use in methadone maintained and untreated intravenous drug users. Drug Alcohol Depend. 1994;36:109-113.

23. Diaz T, Chu SY, Byers RH, Hersh BS, Conti L, Rietmeijer CA, Mokotoff E, Fann A, Boyd D, Iglesias L, Checko PJ, Frederick M, Hermann P, Herr M, Samuel MC. The types of drug used by HIV-infected injection drug users in a multistate surveillance project: Implications for intervention. Am J Public Health. 1994;84:1971-1975.

24. Judson BA, Goldstein A, Inturrisi CE. Methadyl acetate (LAAM) in the treatment of heroin addicts. II. Double-blind comparison of gradual and abrupt detoxification. Arch Gen Psychiatry. 1983;40:834-840.

25. Ling W, Rawson RA, Compton MA. Substitution pharmacotherapies for opioid addiction: From methadone to LAAM and buprenorphine. J Psychoactive Drugs. 1994;26:119-128.

26. Higgins ST, Budney AJ. Treatment of cocaine dependence via the principles of behavioral analysis and behavioral pharmacology. In: Behavioral Treatments for Drug Abuse and Dependence. Proceedings of a meeting. Bethesda, Maryland, September 1-2, 1992. NIDA Res Monogr. 1993;137:97-122.

27. Silverman K, Higgins ST, Brooner RK, et al. Sustained cocaine abstinence in methadone maintenance patients through voucher-based reinforcement therapy. Arch Gen Psychiatry. 1996;53:409-415.

28. Needle RH, Coyle S. Community-based outreach risk-reduction strategy to prevent HIV risk behaviors in out-of-treatment injection drug users. In: NIH Consensus Development Conference, Interventions to Prevent HIV Risk Behaviors. Program and Abstracts, February 11-13, 1997:81-86.

29. Booth R, Crowley, Zhang Y. Substance abuse treatment entry, retention, and effectiveness: Out-of-treatment opiate injection drug users. Drug Alcohol Depend. 1996;42:11-20.

30. Rhodes F, Malotte CK. HIV risk interventions for active drug users: Experience and prospects. In: Oskamp S, Thompson SC (editors). Understanding and Preventing HIV Risk Behavior. Thousand Oaks, CA: Sage Publications, 1996.

31. Jones TS, Haverkos H, Primm B (editors). NIDA/CSAT/CDC workshop on the use of bleach for the decontamination of drug injection equipment (special feature). J Acquir Immune Defic Syndr. 1994;7:741-776.

32. Kaplan EH, Heimer R. HIV incidence among New Haven needle exchange participants: Updated estimates from syringe tracking and testing data. J Acquir Immune Deficiency Syndr. 1995;10:175-176.

33. Hagan H, Des Jarlais DC, Friedman SR, Purchase D, Alter MJ. Reduced risk of hepatitis B and hepatitis C among injection drug users in the Tacoma syringe exchange program. Am J Public Health. 1994;85:1531-1537.

34. Des Jarlais DC. HIV incidence among injecting drug users in New York City Syringe-Exchange Programmes. Lancet. 1996;348:987-991.

35. The White House. The National Drug Control Strategy, 1997. U.S. Government Printing Office, Superintendent of Documents, Mail Stop: SSOP, Washington, DC 20402-9328, 1997.

36. National Institutes of Heath. Consensus Development Conference Statement: Interventions to Prevent HIV Risk Behaviors, February 11-13, 1997.

37. U.S. Department of Health & Human Services. HIV Prevention Bulletin: Medical advice for persons who inject drugs. May 9, 1997.

SELECTIVE GUIDE TO CURRENT REFERENCE SOURCES ON TOPICS DISCUSSED IN THIS ISSUE

Lynn Kasner Morgan, MLS

Each issue of *Journal of Addictive Diseases* features a section offering suggestions on where to look for further information on included topics. The intent is to guide readers to selective substantive sources of current information.

Some published reference works utilize designated terminology (controlled vocabularies) that must be used to find material on topics of interest. For these, a sample of available search terms has been indicated to assist the reader in accessing appropriate sources for his/her purposes. Other reference tools use keywords or free text terms from the title of the document, the abstract, and the name of any responsible agency or conference. In searching using keywords, be sure to look under all possible synonyms to retrieve the concept in question.

An asterisk (*) appearing before a published source indicates that all or part of that source is in machine-readable form and can be accessed through

Lynn Kasner Morgan is Research Associate Professor of Medical Education, Assistant Dean for Information Resources and Systems, and Director of the Gustave L. and Janet W. Levy Library of the Mount Sinai Medical Center, Inc., One Gustave L. Levy Place, New York, NY 10029-6574.

[Haworth co-indexing entry note]: "Selective Guide to Current Reference Sources on Topics Discussed in This Issue." Morgan, Lynn Kasner. Co-published simultaneously in *Journal of Addictive Diseases* (The Haworth Medical Press, an imprint of The Haworth Press, Inc.) Vol. 17, No. 4, 1998, pp. 105-117; and: *Effects of Substance Abuse Treatment on AIDS Risk Behaviors* (ed: Edward Gottheil, and Barry Stimmel) The Haworth Medical Press, an imprint of The Haworth Press, Inc., 1998, pp. 105-117. Single or multiple copies of this article are available for a fee from The Haworth Document Delivery Service [1-800-342-9678, 9:00 a.m. - 5:00 p.m. (EST). E-mail address: getinfo@haworthpressinc.com].

an online database search. Database searching is recommended for retrieving sources of information that coordinate multiple variables, concepts, or subject areas. Most libraries offer database services which can include mediated online searching, access to locally mounted datafiles, front-end software packages, CD-ROM technology and access to the World Wide Web. Searching can also be done from one's office or home with subscriptions to database service vendors and microcomputers equipped with modems.

Interactive electronic communications systems, such as electronic mail, discussion groups, bulletin boards, and receiving and transferring files are available through the Internet, which offers timely and global information resources in all disciplines, including the health sciences. Some groups that might be of interest are: ALCOHOL (ALCOHOL@LMUACAD), DRUG ABUSE (DRUGABUS@UMAB), 12STEP@TRWRB.DSD.COM and ADDIC-TION MEDICINE (MAJORDOMO@AVOCADO.PC.HELSINKI.FI). The National Clearinghouse for Alcohol and Drug Information Center for Substance Abuse Prevention maintains PREVLINE, a bulletin board for alcohol and drug information. Information from PREVLINE is available through the Internet at www.health.org and a recent search included such things as results of the 1997 Monitoring the Future: Survey Data Tables and Figures. There are also many sites with World Wide Web pages which can be reached by individuals with a Web browser such as Microsoft Explorer or Netscape. Netscape "net search" allows searching with many different web search engines. Suggested starting points are http://www.yahoo.com/health, Web Crawler searching tool http://webcrawler.com or idealab's http://www.goto. com. Other sites to try include: Web of Addictions at http://www.well.com/ user/woa; American Psychological Association Division of Pharmacology and Substance Abuse at http://www.apa.org/divisions/div28/index.html; and Online AA resources at http://www.recovery.org. The National Information Services Corporation has made Tobacco and Health Abstracts available on the Web for a fee at http://www.nisc.com. The amount of information available on the Internet increases daily and attention should be given to the author/provider of the information, which ranges from highly respected institutions to individuals with a home computer and a desire to "publish."

Readers are encouraged to consult their librarians for further assistance before undertaking research on a topic.

Suggestions regarding the content and organization of this section are welcome and should be sent to the author.

1. INDEXING AND ABSTRACTING SOURCES

Place of publication, publisher, start date, frequency of publication, and brief descriptions are noted.

Biological Abstracts (1926-) and *Biological Abstracts/RRM* (v. 18, 1980-). Philadelphia, BioSciences Information Service, semimonthly. Reports on worldwide research in the life sciences.

> See: Concept headings for abstracts, such as behavioral biology, pharmacology, psychiatry, public health, and toxicology sections.

> See: Keyword-in-context subject index.

> See Also: http://www.biosis.org

Chemical Abstracts. Columbus, Ohio, American Chemical Society, 1907- , weekly. A key to the world's literature of chemistry and chemical engineering, including serial publications, proceedings and edited collections, technical reports, dissertations, new book and audiovisual materials announcements, and patent documents.

> See: *Index Guide* for cross-referencing and indexing policies.

> See: *General Subject Index* terms, such as drug dependence, drug-drug interactions, drug tolerance.

> See: Keyword subject indexes.

> See Also: http://info.cas.org

Dissertation Abstracts International. Section A. The Humanities and Social Sciences and Section B. The Sciences and Engineering. Ann Arbor, MI, University Microfilms, v.30, 1969/70- , monthly. Includes author-prepared abstracts of doctoral dissertations from 500 participating institutions throughout North America and the world. A separate section contains European dissertations.

> See: Keyword subject index.

> See Also: http://www.umi.com/hp/support/DServices

Excerpta Medica. Amsterdam, The Netherlands, Excerpta Medica Foundation, 1947- , 42 subject sections.

A major abstracting service covering more than 4,300 biomedical journals. The abstracts, including English summaries for non-English-language articles, appear in one or more of the published subject sections, excluding Section 38, *Adverse Reactions Titles,* which is an index only. Each of the sections has a comprehensive subject index. Since 1978 all the *Excerpta Medica* sections have been available for computer searching in the integrated online file, EMBASE. Particularly relevant to the topics in this issue are Section 40, *Drug Dependence, Alcohol Abuse and Alcoholism*; and the sections that have addiction, alcoholism, or drug subdivisions: Section 30, *Clinical and Experimental Pharmacology*; Section 32, *Psychiatry*; and Section 17, *Public Health, Social Medicine and Epidemiology.*

See Also: http://www.excerptamedica.nl

Hospital and Health Administration Index. Chicago, American Hospital Association, v.51, 1995-three issues per year, with annual cumulations. Published as the primary guide to literature on the organization and administration of hospitals and other healthcare providers, the financing and delivery of healthcare, the development and implementation of health policy and reform, and health planning and research.

See: *MeSH* terms, such as acquired immunodeficiency syndrome, alcohol drinking, alcoholism; cocaine; comorbidity; metabolic detoxication, drug; methadone; schizophrenia; substance abuse; substance abuse detection; substance abuse treatment centers; substance dependence; substance withdrawal syndrome.

See Also: http://www.aha.org/resource/hSTAR.html

Index Medicus (includes *Bibliography of Medical Reviews*). Bethesda, MD, National Library of Medicine, 1960- , monthly, with annual cumulations. Published as author and subject indexes to more than 3,000 journals in the biomedical sciences. Subject headings are based on the controlled vocabulary or thesaurus, *Medical Subject Headings (MeSH).* Since 1966 it has been produced from the MEDLARS database, which provides more comprehensive retrieval, including keyword access and English-language abstracts, than its printed counterparts:

Index Medicus, International Nursing Index, and *Index to Dental Literature.*

See: *MeSH* terms, such as acquired immunodeficiency syndrome, cocaine, comorbidity; metabolic detoxification, drug; methadone; analgesics opiod; substance abuse; substance abuse treatment centers; substance dependence; substance withdrawal syndrome.

See Also: http://www.ncbi.nlm.nih.gov/PubMed

http://igm.nlm.nih.gov

Index to Scientific Reviews. Philadelphia, Institute for Scientific Information, 1974- , semiannual.

See: Permuterm keyword subject index.

See: Citation index.

*International Pharmaceutical Abstracts. Washington, DC, American Society of Health-System Pharmacists, 1964- , semimonthly. A key to the world's literature of pharmacy.

See: IPA subject terms, such as cocaine; controlled substances; dependence; drug abuse; drug withdrawal; methadone; opiates; pharmacotherapy.

See: Subject sections: legislation, laws and regulations; sociology, economics and ethics; toxicology.

See Also: http://www.dialog.com

*Psychological Abstracts. Washington, DC, American Psychological Association, 1927- , monthly. A compilation of nonevaluative summaries of the world's literature in psychology and related disciplines.

See: Index terms, such as acquired immune deficiency syndrome; cocaine; addiction; comorbidity; drug abuse; drug addiction; drug dependency; drug rehabilitation; drug therapy; drug usage; drug withdrawal; methadone; opiates; social issues; psychopharmacology; treatment outcomes.

See Also: http://www.apa.org/psychnet

*Public Affairs Information Service Bulletin. New York, Public Affairs Information Service, v.55, 1969- , semimonthly. An index to library material in the field of public affairs and public policy published throughout the world.

See: PAIS subject headings, such as cocaine; drug abuse; drug addicts; drugs.

See Also: http://www.pais.inter.net

Science Citation Index. Philadelphia, Institute for Scientific Information, 1961- , bimonthly.

See: Permuterm keyword subject index.

See: Citation index.

See Also: http://www.isinet.com

Social Work Abstracts. New York, National Association of Social Workers, v.13, 1977- , quarterly.

See: Subject index.

See Also: http://www.naswdc.org

Sociological Abstracts. San Diego, CA, Sociological Abstracts, Inc., 1952- , 6 times per year. A collection of nonevaluative abstracts which reflect the world's serial literature in sociology and related disciplines.

See: *Thesaurus of Sociological Indexing Terms.*

See: Descriptors such as acquired immune deficiency syndrome; addict/addicts/addicted/addictive/addiction; cocaine; detoxification; drug abuse; drug addiction; drug use; habits; methadone maintenance; substance abuse.

See Also: http://www.accessinn.com/socabs

2. CURRENT AWARENESS PUBLICATIONS

Current Contents: Clinical Medicine. Philadelphia, Institute for Scientific Information, v.15, 1987- , weekly.

See: Keyword index.

See Also: http://www.isinet.com

Current Contents: Life Sciences. Philadelphia, Institute for Scientific Information, v.10, 1967- , weekly.

See: Keyword index.

See Also: http://www.isinet.com

Current Contents: Social & Behavioral Sciences. Philadelphia, Institute for Scientific Information, v.6, 1974- , weekly.

See: Keyword index.

See Also: http://www.isinet.com

3. BOOKS

Medical and Health Care Books and Serials in Print: An Index to Literature in the Health Sciences. New York, R. R. Bowker Co., annual.

See: Library of Congress subject headings, such as drug abuse; drugs; cocaine; methadone maintenance; narcotic habit; pharmacology; substance abuse.

Bellenir, Karen. *Substance Abuse Sourcebook.* Detroit, Omnigraphics, 1996.

O'Brien, Robert [and others]. *The Encyclopedia of Drug Abuse.* 2nd ed. New York, Facts on File, c1992.

Stimmel, Barry [and others]. *The Facts About Drug Use: Coping with Drug Use in Your Family, at Work, in Your Community.* Mount Vernon, N.Y., Consumers Union, c1991.

Substance Abuse: The Nation's Number One Health Problem, Key Indicators for Policy. Princeton, NJ, Robert Wood Johnson Foundation, 1993.

Kinney, Jean. *Clinical Manual of Substance Abuse.* St. Louis, Mosby, 1996.

World Health Organization Catalogue: New Books. Geneva, World Health Organization, semiannual (supplements *World Health Organization Publications* and includes periodicals).

See Also: http://www.who.org

4. U.S. GOVERNMENT PUBLICATIONS

Alcohol and Other Drug Thesaurus: A Guide to Concepts and Terminology in Substance Abuse and Addiction (AOD Thesaurus). Rockville, MD, National Institute on Alcohol Abuse and Alcoholism, 2nd ed., 1995.

See: Title keyword index.

See Also: http://www.niaaa.nih.gov

Monthly Catalog of United States Government Publications. Washington, DC, U.S. Government Printing Office, 1895- , monthly.

See: Keyword index.

See Also: http://www.access.gpo.gov

5. ONLINE BIBLIOGRAHIC DATABASES

Only those databases that have no print counterparts are included in this section. Print sources that have online database equivalents are noted throughout this guide by the asterisk (*) which appears before the title. If you do not have direct access to these databases, consult your librarian for assistance.

ALCOHOL AND ALCOHOL PROBLEMS SCIENCE DATABASE: ETOH (National Institute on Alcohol Abuse and Alcoholism, Rockville, MD).

Use: Keywords.

See Also: http://etoh.niaaa.nih.gov

ALCOHOL INFORMATION FOR CLINICIANS AND EDUCATORS (Project Cork Institute, Dartmouth Medical School, Hanover, NH).

Use: Keywords.

See Also: http://www.dartmouth.edu/dms/cork

AMERICAN STATISTICS INDEX (ASI) (Congressional Information Services, Inc., Washington, DC).

Use: Keywords.

DRUG INFORMATION FULLTEXT (American Society of Health-System Pharmacists, Bethesda, MD).

Use: Keywords.

DRUGINFO AND ALCOHOL USE AND ABUSE (Hazelden Foundation, Center City, MN, and Drug Information Service Center, College of Pharmacy, University of Minnesota, Minneapolis, MN).

> Use: Keywords.

> See Also: http://www.hazelden.org

LEXIS (LEXIS–NEXIS, Dayton, OH).

> Use: Guide library.

> See Also: http://www.lexis-nexis.com

MAGAZINE DATABASE (Information Access Co., Foster City, CA).

> Use: Keywords.

> See Also: http://www.informationaccess.com

MENTAL HEALTH ABSTRACTS (MHA) (IFI/Plenum Data Co., Wilmington, NC).

> Use: Keywords.

> See Also: http://www.ifiplenum.com/mhainf.htm

NATIONAL NEWSPAPER INDEX (Information Access Co., Foster City, CA).

> Use: Keywords.

NTIS (Bibliographic Data Base, U.S. National Technical Information Service, Springfield, VA).

> Use: Keywords.

> See Also: http://www.ntis.gov

PSYCINFO (American Psychological Association, Washington, DC).

> Use: Keywords.

See Also: http://www.apa.org/psychnet

WESTLAW (West Publishing Co., Eagan, MN).

Use: Keywords.

See Also: http://www.westgroup.com

6. HANDBOOKS, DIRECTORIES, GRANT SOURCES, ETC.

Annual Register of Grant Support. Wilamette, IL, National Register Pub. Co., annual.

See: Internal medicine; medicine; pharmacology, psychiatry, psychology, mental health sections.

See: Subject index.

*Biomedical Index to PHS-Supported Research. Bethesda, MD, National Institutes of Health, Division of Research Grants, annual.

See: Subject index.

Directory of Research Grants. Phoenix, AR, Oryx Press, annual.

See: Subject index terms, such as education, drugs/drug abuse, health promotion.

*Encyclopedia of Associations. Detroit, Gale Research Co., annual (occasional supplements between editions).

See: Subject index.

*Foundation Directory. New York, The Foundation Center, biennial (updated between editions by *Foundation Directory Supplement*).

See: Index of foundations.

See: Index of foundations by state and city.

See: Index of donors, trustees, and administrators.

See: Index of fields of interest.

See Also: http://www.fdncenter.org

Health Hotlines: Toll-Free Numbers from DIRLINE. Bethesda, MD, National Library of Medicine, biennial.

Information Industry Directory. Detroit, Gale Research Co., annual.

Nolan, Kathleen Lopez. *Gale Directory of Databases.* Detroit, Gale Research, Inc., annual.

Roper, Fred W. and Jo Anne Boorkman. *Introduction to Reference Sources in the Health Sciences.* 3rd ed. Chicago, Medical Library Association, c1994.

Statistics Sources. 22nd ed. Detroit, Gale Research Inc., annual.

7. JOURNAL LISTINGS

The Serials Directory. An International Reference Book. Birmingham, Ebsco Publishing, annual (supplemented by quarterly updates).

Ulrich's International Periodicals Directory, Now Including Irregular Serials & Annuals. New York, R. R. Bowker Co., annual (updated between editions by *Ulrich's Quarterly*).

See: Subject categories, such as drug abuse and alcoholism, medical sciences, pharmacy and pharmacology, psychology, public health and safety.

8. AUDIOVISUAL PROGRAMS

The Directory of Medical Video Programs. Hawthorne, NJ, Ridge Publishing Co., 1990.

National Library of Medicine Audiovisuals Catalog. Bethesda, MD, National Library of Medicine, 1977-1993, quarterly, with annual cumulations.

See: *MeSH* terms as noted in Section 1 under *Index Medicus*.

Patient Education Sourcebook. 2v. Saint Louis, MO, Health Sciences Communications Association, c1985-90.

See: *MeSH* terms as noted in Section 1 under *Index Medicus.*

9. GUIDES TO UPCOMING MEETINGS

Scientific Meetings. San Diego, CA, Scientific Meetings Publications, quarterly.

See: Subject indexes.

See: Association listing.

World Meetings: Medicine. New York, Macmillan Pub. Co., quarterly.

See: Keyword index.

See: Sponsor directory and index.

World Meetings: Social and Behavioral Sciences, Human Services and Management. New York, Macmillan Pub. Co., quarterly.

See: Keyword index.

See: Sponsor directory and index.

10. PROCEEDINGS OF MEETINGS

*Directory of Published Proceedings. Series SEMT. Science/Engineering/Medicine/Technology. Harrison, NY, InterDok Corp., v.3, 1967- , monthly, except July-August, with annual cumulations.

See: http://www.interdok.com

*Index to Scientific and Technical Proceedings. Philadelphia, Institute for Scientific Information, 1978- , monthly with semiannual cumulations.

See: htpp://www.isinet.com

11. SPECIALIZED RESEARCH CENTERS

Medical Research Centres. Harlow, Essex, Longman, biennial.

International Research Centers Directory. Detroit, Gale Research Co., annual.

Research Centers Directory. Detroit, Gale Research Co., annual (updated by *New Research Centers*).

12. SPECIAL LIBRARY COLLECTIONS

Directory of Special Libraries and Information Centers. Detroit, Gale Research Co., annual (updated by *New Special Libraries*).

Index

Abstinence, from stimulant abuse, 29
Acquaintances, as drug use
    companions, 14,15,16,17
Acquired immunodeficiency
    syndrome (AIDS). *See also*
    Human immunodeficiency
    virus (HIV) entries
    as mortality cause, 50
    rates of, 92-94
Acquired immunodeficiency
    syndrome cases, numbers of
    annual, 92
    total, 34
    worldwide, 1
Addiction Severity Index
    description of, 36
    scores on
        of outpatient drug treatment
        patients, 64,65
        relationship to psychiatric
        disorder comorbidity,
        36,38,40,42
        effect on stimulant abuse
        treatment on, 24-25
Adolescents, sexually-transmitted
    AIDS cases among, 20
Africa, HIV/AIDS epidemic in, 92
African Americans
    HIV/AIDS prevalence in, 92,93
    sexually-transmitted AIDS cases
    among, 20
AIDS Knowledge Survey scores, of
    outpatient drug treatment
    patients, 64,65,66-67
AIDS Risk Inventory (AR-I), 55-57
Alcohol use, as HIV risk, 86,93-94
    databases regarding, 112
    among homosexual/bisexual males,
    23,92

among methadone-maintained
    cocaine users,
    75,76-77,78,83,84,86
among outpatient drug treatment
    patients, 65,66
AMERICAN STATISTICS INDEX,
    112
Amphetamine use
    by intravenous drug users, 95-96
    as sexually-transmitted HIV risk,
    21
    among homosexuals, 92
Antisocial personality disorder,
    3,35,45,83-84,86-87
Asia, HIV/AIDs prevalence in, 92
Assessment instruments, for drug
    abuse-related HIV
    transmission, 49-59
    assessment domains of, 53-55
Audiovisual programs, 115-116

"Backloading," 10
Baltimore, drug treatment programs
    in, 2
Beck Depression Inventory
    description of, 37
    scores on
        of outpatient drug treatment
        patients, 64,65
        relationship to psychiatric
        disorder comorbidity,
        37,40,41,42,43,44
Behavioral therapy
    for cocaine addiction, 96
    for HIV infection prevention, 5
Bibliographic databases,
    105-106,112-114,115
Biological Abstracts, 107

    119

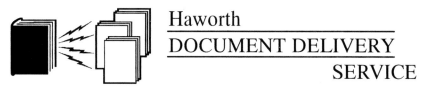

Haworth
DOCUMENT DELIVERY
SERVICE

This valuable service provides a single-article order form for any article from a Haworth journal.

- *Time Saving:* No running around from library to library to find a specific article.
- *Cost Effective:* All costs are kept down to a minimum.
- *Fast Delivery:* Choose from several options, including same-day FAX.
- *No Copyright Hassles:* You will be supplied by the original publisher.
- *Easy Payment:* Choose from several easy payment methods.

Open Accounts Welcome for ...
- Library Interlibrary Loan Departments
- Library Network/Consortia Wishing to Provide Single-Article Services
- Indexing/Abstracting Services with Single Article Provision Services
- Document Provision Brokers and Freelance Information Service Providers

MAIL or *FAX* THIS ENTIRE ORDER FORM TO:

Haworth Document Delivery Service
The Haworth Press, Inc.
10 Alice Street
Binghamton, NY 13904-1580

or FAX: 1-800-895-0582
or CALL: 1-800-429-6784
9am-5pm EST

PLEASE SEND ME PHOTOCOPIES OF THE FOLLOWING SINGLE ARTICLES:
1) Journal Title: _____
   Vol/Issue/Year: _____ Starting & Ending Pages: _____
   Article Title: _____

2) Journal Title: _____
   Vol/Issue/Year: _____ Starting & Ending Pages: _____
   Article Title: _____

3) Journal Title: _____
   Vol/Issue/Year: _____ Starting & Ending Pages: _____
   Article Title: _____

4) Journal Title: _____
   Vol/Issue/Year: _____ Starting & Ending Pages: _____
   Article Title: _____

(See other side for Costs and Payment Information)

COSTS: Please figure your cost to order quality copies of an article.

1. Set-up charge per article: $8.00
   ($8.00 × number of separate articles) _____

2. Photocopying charge for each article:
   1-10 pages: $1.00 _____

   11-19 pages: $3.00 _____

   20-29 pages: $5.00 _____

   30+ pages: $2.00/10 pages _____

3. Flexicover (optional): $2.00/article _____

4. Postage & Handling: US: $1.00 for the first article/
   $.50 each additional article _____

   Federal Express: $25.00 _____

   Outside US: $2.00 for first article/
   $.50 each additional article _____

5. Same-day FAX service: $.50 per page _____

GRAND TOTAL: _____

METHOD OF PAYMENT: (please check one)

❑ Check enclosed ❑ Please ship and bill. PO # _____
   (sorry we can ship and bill to bookstores only! All others must pre-pay)

❑ Charge to my credit card: ❑ Visa; ❑ MasterCard; ❑ Discover;
   ❑ American Express;

Account Number: _____ Expiration date: _____

Signature: *X* _____

Name: _____ Institution: _____

Address: _____

_____

City: _____ State: _____ Zip: _____

Phone Number: _____ FAX Number: _____

MAIL or *FAX* THIS ENTIRE ORDER FORM TO:

Haworth Document Delivery Service	**or FAX:** 1-800-895-0582
The Haworth Press, Inc.	**or CALL:** 1-800-429-6784
10 Alice Street	(9am-5pm EST)
Binghamton, NY 13904-1580	